BECOMING IMMORTAL

Nanotechnology, You, and the Demise of Death

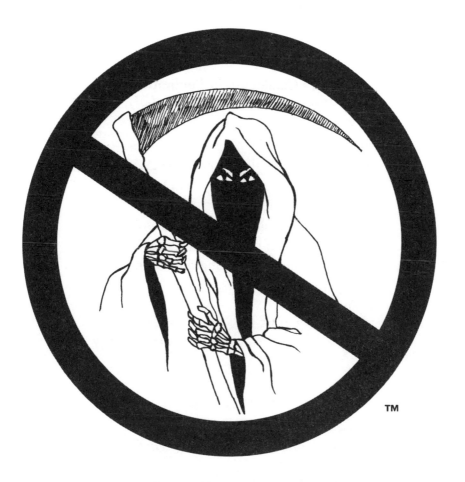

™

Wesley M. Du Charme, Ph.D.

BECOMING IMMORTAL
Copyright © 1995 by Wesley M. DuCharme
All rights reserved.

Blue Creek Ventures
P.O. Box 3266
Evergreen, CO 80439

First Edition

Publisher's Cataloging-in-Publication Data
(Prepared by Quality Books Inc.)

DuCharme, Wesley M.
    Becoming immortal: nanotechnology, you, and the
demise of death / by Wesley M. DuCharme.
    p. cm.
    Includes bibliographical references and index.
    ISBN 0-9646282-0-1   LCC 95-94347
    1. Nanotechnology. 2. Longevity. 3. Immortalism.
    4. Cryonics.
    I. Title
    T174.7.D83 1995   620.4
                                       QBI95-20187

Book Design by:
Dianne J. Borneman
Shadow Canyon Graphics, Evergreen, Colorado

Printed in the United States of America

Contents

Acknowledgements

I am much indebted to the people who discussed, argued, encouraged, snorted at, and generally helped me shape the ideas contained in this book. To Steve Bridge, Chris Butler, Skippy Du Charme, Jack Fleming, Nicole Fussell, Bonnie Neighbors, Liz Netzel, Bert Newman, Mike and Lynn Noel, Chris Peterson, Don Wargo and Paul Weaver—my sincere thanks.

I would also like to apologize to Steven B. Harris for stealing his very amusing title to head up Chapter 17. You will find the looted article listed under his name in the reference section.

It will be obvious to those familiar with his works that much of what this book contains is based on the pioneering, awe-inspiring creativity of K. Eric Drexler. Neither he nor anyone listed above, though, is to blame for any mistakes or errors in this book. They can take the bows; I'll take the flak.

For my wife Skippy—my immortal beloved.

BEGINNINGS

> I don't want to achieve
> immortality through
> my work.
> I want to achieve it
> through not dying.
>
> Woody Allen

Let's clear the air, here.
You read the title and decided to
crack the book open for a second,
but you're way past skeptical.
If I give you the slightest excuse,
you'll put this book down
like a shot and get on with
your respectable, rational life.
So, why don't we talk about your fears?

CHAPTER 1

Top Ten Reasons Not To Read This Book

1. I figure this is some tricky way to get me to read a religious tome about how I can attain life everlasting in the bosom of the Lord.

Not so. This is a book about what's possible right here and now—in this world.

2. OK, so it's a trick to get me to read a book about how to eat right and exercise and lead a disgustingly healthy life.

Wrong. Those aren't bad ideas, but they have very little to do with what will be discussed here.

3. I gave your intentions the benefit of a doubt, but now I'm getting suspicious. You're probably some kind of charlatan trying to push a miracle drug or elixir of ground-up monkey glands.

Dead wrong...you should pardon the expression.

4. Well, even the last one gave you some credit for rationality, though I thought you were trying to take advantage of me. Now we're reduced to pure quackery. You must have gone 'round the bend and want me to follow you.

Possible I guess, I'd probably be the last one to know, but I think my ducks are all in a line. In any case, you'll see that the ideas discussed in this book have lots of support and didn't spring full-blown from my lonely brain. I'm mostly pulling together and summarizing concepts and developments that are talked about other places by other people.

5. All right, if you're not crazy and you're not trying to sell me some exotic death-defying product, then you must be doing this just to sell books.

Well, not 'just,' but that's not a bad motive in a capitalistic society, right? I do have other reasons, though. This book is full of positive, hopeful information I think you'd like to know about. And the more of us who know about the exciting prospects, and talk about them, the more likely good things are to happen. That's just the way the world works.

6. OK, OK, your motives are relatively pure, and you're actually going to talk about what the book title suggests you're going to talk about. Then I have a truly serious problem because it just ain't possible, so no point spending my money and time on the book.

Wrong yet again, dear reader. It is possible, and there's no reason why it can't happen, why you can't be immortal.

7. Sure, uh huh, anything is possible. A million monkeys hammering away at computer keyboards might churn out a passable plan for balancing the federal budget (although present evidence suggests the contrary). That doesn't mean it's going to happen anytime in the foreseeable future, for sure not in my lifetime.

On "foreseeable future" I'd have to disagree with you. Regarding "in your lifetime," your chances depend in part on how old you are, how many times you go hang gliding a week and such things. But, let's say you're right and it's not in your lifetime. Still, there's a strategy that can get you from here to there. Kind of high tech, maybe a little crazy sounding at first, but you *do* want to live forever, right?

8. So, for the sake of argument, I'll allow that immortality is possible. It might become possible in my lifetime, or something magical might extend my lifetime until it does become possible. But, now that I think about it, immortality is probably not a very good damn idea anyway. People living forever — we're already overcrowded and polluted, ruining the planet, running short of resources. So even if I could do it, I probably shouldn't.

Wrong for nearly the last time. The book offers you two words to allay those fears, to soothe those concerns. The words are "molecular nanotechnology". Whoa! Two words, eleven syllables. Fetch the smelling salts, Martha.

9. The title is either hokey or sensationalistic; the tone of the book, as evidenced so far by this list, doesn't really sound very serious; and my leg is probably going to get severely yanked.

Your leg may get yanked, but not by me. I'm serious, and so are the other people writing about and working on the concepts to be discussed. After all, what could be more serious than the topic of death? But what you see (so far) is what you get. There's no reason not to have fun as we explore these fascinating ideas, is there? Hey, it's not life-or-death, it's life-instead-of-death. Anyway, there will be plenty of references of a more serious, technical nature cited if you want to dig deeper.

10. The book costs too much money, and my brother-in-law won't lend me his copy. He doesn't believe my story about the black hole that ate all the other books he lent me.

Narrow-minded bugger, isn't he? Try the library.

CHAPTER 2

Death's Demise:
Getting the Word Out

> Neither in the hearts of men
> nor in the manners of society
> will there be a lasting peace
> until we outlaw death.
>
> Albert Camus

Have I dealt with some of those pesky doubts of yours? Well, here you are in Chapter 2, so let's get on with things.

The central thesis of this book is that there are practical steps you can take which will lead to physical immortality. The book will lead you gently through the whole story and show you how to accomplish each step.

9

Exactly what do you mean by "physical immortality"?

Just what it sounds like. You, in your very own body, with all your memories, surviving down the ages. Strictly speaking, *immortal* means living forever, and if one should "never say never," one probably should "forever avoid forever."

One of the most popular current theories of the origin and destination of the universe suggests that it started with a big bang and will someday collapse down to a vanishingly small point and then, perhaps, start all over again. It's not likely that anything will survive that collapse, but it also won't happen for billions of years. That's close enough to forever for me, but you're allowed to quibble if you want. We'll talk more about "true" immortality in a later chapter.

If people can become immortal, why haven't I heard anything about it?

Good question to which I'm not sure I know the answer. First, let me state that there are a fair number of people who *do* know about the prospects for immortality, so it's not like a great secret is being revealed here for the very first time right before your eyes.

So that the book doesn't come across as one big tease, let me cite some sources for you right now. The most complete nuts-and-bolts treatment of the topic is in K.

Eric Drexler's *Engines of Creation* (1986). Reference to key concepts can also be found in *Unbounding the Future* (1991) and in *Cryonics: Reaching for Tomorrow* (1993).

Complete references to these works and others can be found at the back of the book. My intention in this book is to explain the concepts in a non-technical way and to give you practical advice on steps that you can take towards achieving immortality.

So, same question. If there is some practical means for me to achieve immortality, why isn't it plastered all over the newspapers, covered on the 10 o'clock news, discussed ad nauseam on the talk shows?

Well, we've established that it's not a state secret, so there must be some other explanation. I'll list a few likely candidates:

- disbelief
- intellectual inertia
- religion
- technological ignorance/trauma
- future shock
- lack of imagination
- fear of change
- fear of disappointment
- fear of being thought weird, crazy, obsessed, inappropriate

- and, maybe the biggest one, unwillingness to contemplate death.

Let's talk about the last one. Contemplating immortality necessarily means contemplating mortality, and there seems to be something about humans which makes it difficult for them to do that. Oh, sure, everyone thinks about death now and then—why else would wills be written and burial plots be sold? But death is not a pleasant thought, and no one, other than the mentally ill, makes the contemplation a full-time occupation.

Disbelief enters here, too. If one really thought there was a viable alternative, perhaps thinking about death wouldn't be so bad. But, virtually no one thinks there is a viable alternative. Catch 22. You can't avoid death because you refuse to think about it.

So, what's a poor mortal to do?

Keep reading.

Being thought crazy or obsessed can also be a big deterrent. Of course inventors from Galileo to the Wright brothers have been viewed that way. Your advantage is that you don't have to invent the technology, just use it. Still, you will probably be viewed as odd at best if you start bragging to the guys in the bar that you're planning to make Methuselah look like a mayfly pantywaist.

> If you live to the age of a
> hundred you have it made
> because very few people die
> past the age of a hundred.
>
> George Burns

It is hard to think of a concept more firmly rooted in our lives than that of death. The line that goes "there are only two sure things in life, death and taxes" uses death as the ironic counterpoint to taxes for good reason. In fact, for any individual, the only two certainties are birth and death. Everything in between is subject to negotiation. What could loom larger in the minds of self-aware beings than their own dissolution? There are some who

> Death is the source of
> meaning. If you could live
> forever, life would be
> meaningless. Death is the
> source of man. There is no
> self without death.
>
> (in Smith, 1983)

feel that life cannot be defined without the concept of death attached to it, just as goodness needs evil to help define it.

The ingrained nature of that way of viewing life makes the concept of immortality difficult to grasp. In fact, many people exhibit a knee-jerk rejection of the concept once it is seriously introduced. Clearly, that is one of the many mental obstacles you will face in considering that death may have a demise.

Chapter 3

The Mental Obstacle Course

> There is nothing either
> good or bad, but thinking
> makes it so.
>
> William Shakespeare

You have a chance to become physically immortal—and there are things you can do to make that chance a reasonably good one. That, in a nutshell, is the thesis of this book.

I believe the most serious obstacle you'll have to overcome in order to have a chance at physical immortality is the obstacle presented by a mind-set which says it is not possible. If you can withhold judgment long enough to let some new information seep in, if you can open-mindedly evaluate some arguments and evidence, you may have a chance.

This book has two main sections, "Arguments Against Immortality" and "How To Get From Here To There". The rest of this introduction will be devoted to convincing you that there is good reason for you to keep reading rather than dismissing the idea of immortality out of hand.

> New opinions are always
> suspected, and usually
> opposed, without any other
> reason but because they are
> not already common.
>
> John Locke

You'll find that the key element of the discussions of immortality, the arguments that make immortality plausible to at least some people, have to do with advances in technology—advances which are foreseeable from where we are in the present. The ability of humans to make accurate predictions of future advances in technology thus becomes of paramount importance to the discussion.

If you have some problem with the concept of immortality which does not relate to its possibility and would like to jump to that concern, I invite you to go to the section covering "Arguments Against Immortality" and see what is said regarding your number one doubt or concern. Maybe your concern will be relieved or at least put in abeyance, and maybe not. You might as well start, though, with whatever makes you think immortality is a bad or stupid idea. You can always come back to here, or jump to wherever in the book you want. Whatever you do, give the book— and yourself—a fair chance.

The book promises to tell you how to achieve immortality. My readings and discussions with a variety of people about the concept suggest that your biggest problem will be in overcoming your skepticism that immortality is even remotely possible. If you can get past that skepticism, the rest of the process is not so difficult to bring about. You'll see that there is a logical flow to the arguments presented. The arguments are based on current technology and reasonable projections of the capabilities of future technology. I think you will find that each step in the argument is plausible. When the whole sequence is put together, you will find you have arrived at obviously startling conclusions having to do with extreme longevity, or what most people would call immortality.

Still skeptical? Consider this question. How likely is it that, right now, you have a good understanding of what the possibilities are for attaining physical immortality? I would argue that the chances depend on two things: first your knowledge of advances taking place in a variety of scientific and technological disciplines, and second your ability to extrapolate or predict from that knowledge base to what is likely to happen in the future. If you are knowledgeable in the proper disciplines and can make good extrapolations, your understanding of our chances for attaining physical immortality will be correspondingly good. Conversely, if you fall short in either of these areas your understanding will be faulty.

The hard part, perhaps surprisingly, is not attaining the knowledge. Many people have the capability of reading enough, learning enough, knowing enough. The problem is in taking that knowledge and accurately extrapolating it. My Ph.D. thesis, some years back, had that as its subject. I attempted to experimentally determine why humans are conservative when taking in new information and revising their opinion about something. I haven't been involved in that field of study for some years, but research is still finding that experts and non-experts alike have a large "surprise index" when they estimate probabilities (Cooke, 1991). That is, there are large differences between the estimated and actual probabilities.

However, you don't need to look at what some would consider arcane psychological research to understand the point. History is replete with famous examples of incorrect assessments of evidence leading to wrong predictions. New ideas just have a tough time making it in the world. A few examples:

- The germ theory of disease was put forward by Joseph Lister in 1865. Thirty years later physicians were still operating without masks or head coverings.

- Various forms of anesthesia were available beginning as early as 1846. Some physicians, however, thought pain during surgery was simply natural and inevitable.

- Orville and Wilbur lifted off from Kittyhawk in 1903. "Yet for five years, Washington didn't believe that the Wright brothers had actually flown—because everybody knew it was impossible. Leading scientists were then still writing papers proving it couldn't be done." (Clarke, 1994). Once it was proven possible, the United States military did not believe that airplanes were of any strategic value other than as observation platforms.

- Lord Rutherford, the famous British physicist, ten years before the first atomic bomb exploded, was of the opinion that there could be no practical applications of atomic energy. You might say his opinion bombed.

- In 1977, Ernst Chain, the co-discoverer of penicillin, said: "There exists no method, at present, nor is there likelihood that one will be discovered in the foreseeable future, by which it would be possible...to alter...the genetic properties in any gene of any mammalian cell in a controlled manner which could be called 'genetic engineering'". Twelve years later genes were being delivered to specific positions in the DNA of animals.

- Travel by space ship to other planets was long relegated to the realm of "mere science fiction" (more about that later). In 1956 the Astronomer Royal of Britain gave his opinion that "Space travel is utter bilge." Thirteen years later we landed on the moon. Indeed, many people did not believe space travel would ever occur and I've read of people who *still* think it hasn't happened, that it's all a hoax perpetrated by NASA or some other group. The only kind of travel to the moon they believe in is the kind provided by Ralph Kramden (of Honeymooner's fame).

Please note—we're not only talking about the man in the street here, we're also talking about experts in the field. They had the knowledge base, but lacked the ability to make accurate forecasts based on the knowledge. I mention this not to find fault, but to make the point again that accurately revising one's opinion as new data become available is not something that humans do particularly well.

> ...because people, thought to be realistic, only
> believe developments are likely when they are
> nearly upon us, the time we have to think about
> what to do with the
> discoveries is usually much too short.
>
> Johathan Glover

Of course, citing examples where forecasts of technology were notoriously wrong shows only part of the picture. Conservative predictions which proved right receive much less notice or interest and are undoubtedly more common. Where immortality is concerned, however, I suggest that conservative opinions be examined very closely—as though your life depended on it.

So, what makes me and others like me, who believe in the possibility of immortality, think that we know how to predict the technology of the future? Well, maybe we don't. But we're aware of the innate conservatism of humans in this area. We're also aware that once certain things are in place, progress in a given field seems inevitable. For now, let's turn to another factor that may have a distorting effect on the way you process information relating to the possibility of immortality.

Most people hate to think or talk about their own deaths. Everyone comes to grips with it one way or

> **Man is the only animal that
> knows it is going to die.**
>
> **Philip Wylie**

another; but once they have worked their way through the issue, perhaps by deciding to ignore it as much as possible, they prefer Pandora's box to remain closed. It is not a comfortable issue to deal with.

Among the more basic comforts people get from religion is the thought of an afterlife. They find comfort in the thought that when they die, their story does not end in what a friend of mine calls "the big dirt nap." Even so, they are not likely to dwell on their own dissolution, no matter how happy they think their next life may be.

> **Death is just a distant rumor to the young.**
>
> **Andy Rooney**

It is often observed that young people act as though they were immortal. They take chances most adults avoid. In their case, chance taking is probably less a denial of death than it is an inability to even conceive of it.

Death is the flip side of the coin on which immortality is stamped. If you can't stand thinking about one, it will be hard to contemplate the other. Conversely, if you can't entertain notions of immortality, death will remain the sure thing it has always been down all the ages...the coin will never flip.

Now that we've talked about some general factors that may get in your way when thinking about immortality and evaluating information, let's move on to more specific arguments.

ARGUMENTS

AGAINST

IMMORTALITY

CHAPTER 4

The Plausibility Hurdle

> And death shall have no dominion.
>
> Dylan Thomas

Who, in their right mind, would believe in the possibility of physical immortality?

A number of otherwise seemingly rational people, perhaps even including you by the time you get through reading this book, believe in the possibility of immortality. From a logical point of view, overcoming the plausibility hurdle is the single most important task of this book. If you can't get past this question, none of the other arguments against immortality need be considered. So, plausibility is where we will begin.

The argument starts with the notion that your body is a machine, a biological machine. A corollary of this argument is that you, the 'you' we're going to talk about preserving, *are* your body including your brain and the information contained in it. The reasoning is that information—the information encoded in your brain including your memories and personality factors—constitutes the essential you.

The more philosophically inclined may notice that I am skipping over a lot of debate on just what constitutes consciousness, how self-identity is determined, and other such questions. Since this is a practical book, oriented toward the technologically possible, the reader will have to look elsewhere if those less concrete things are of concern. On the matter of a "soul," for instance, I think most people would accept the argument that as long as the body is functioning the soul will remain attached. Therefore, I assume that when I discuss what might happen with your body, less physical matters need not be of concern.

You are a machine, you break down. You are a very complex biological machine that has self-repair mechanisms built in—and those mechanisms work pretty well most of the time. As you age, however, they stop working so well, and eventually they fail altogether. Parts fail, systems fail, you die. However, machines can be repaired. Your body can be repaired—and if you're like me it probably has been.

For centuries medical science has been discovering ways to make repairs, ways to help your body survive damage. These repair techniques vary in sophistication. At one end are the crudities of limb amputation aimed at stopping the spread of an infection, and at the other, very modern high technology gene therapy techniques in which special genes are inserted to compensate for some genetic defect, such as being born with a faulty immune system. In between are preventative measures such as maintaining the proper amount of vitamins and minerals in your body. (An old example is making sure you have enough vitamin C to prevent scurvy.)

> There are no such things as incurables.
> There are only things for which man has
> not found a cure.
>
> **Bernard Baruch**

Medical science is making advances on an almost daily basis aimed at repairing the ravages of disease, age, genetic defects, and a multitude of other problems. In November, 1993, for instance, the American Medical Association published over 150 articles in eleven medical journals on the topic of molecular genetics. One could argue on the basis of that kind of progress that eventually people will be immortal, or nearly so—that aging will be cured. There is nothing in principle to suggest otherwise. It is true at this point that there *seems* to be some naturally occurring limit to the age a human can reach. One possible interpretation of that fact is simply that, so far, we can't repair the machine once it reaches such a point. It doesn't mean that we'll *never* be able to repair it.

But, the steady march of medical progress could leave us centuries or thousands of years away from the ability to repair and maintain the human machine in prime condition. In fact, immortality is not seen as a goal by many. Both the difficulty of achieving immortality and the perceived nature of the problems it might bring serve to dampen enthusiasm. Happily, recent developments in a new, interdisciplinary area of scientific endeavor called nanotechnology promise to bring the vague hope of immortality—sometime—much more sharply, and quickly, into focus.

The path to a future where the human machine can be repaired and maintained at the cellular level was first laid out by K. Eric Drexler in the previously referenced *Engines of Creation* in 1986. The explanation of nanotechnology which follows draws heavily from that source and other Drexler publications.

So, what exactly is nanotechnology?

The term was invented by Drexler and appears in *Engines of Creation*. It refers to physical operations carried out at the nanometer level (one billionth of a meter). The basis of the technology is the mechanical assembly of molecules to build complex structures.

Drexler essentially took strands from a number of separate areas of scientific endeavor including chemistry, genetic engineering, physics and computer science and wove them together into a single new strand which he calls nanotechnology.

Drexler earned, from the Massachusetts Institute of Technology, the first-ever Ph.D. in nanotechnology. He has taught the subject at Stanford and other universities and leads the nanotechnology movement. Since his coining of the term, nanotechnology has been applied more broadly than was his original intent. He now refers to his concept as *molecular nanotechnology* and to the application of the technology as *molecular manufacturing*. For the sake of simplicity I will continue to refer to it as simply "nanotechnology."

The essence of nanotechnology is control of matter at the molecular level, that is, the manipulation of molecules to build desired structures. The kind of engineering envisioned has *structures being built molecule by molecule with complete positional control of each molecule so as to arrive at the desired structure*. Those simple words lead to a sweeping, fundamental, awesome change in the way humans will live. The technology will change the degree of control we have over our world, over the manufacturing process, over the creation of foodstuff, and over our own bodies.

This is not a technical book about nanotechnology (several of those exist), but rather a nontechnical look at the enormous possibilities that lie before us, in particular as they relate to human immortality. Those wishing the technical details are referred to Drexler's books and the other sources mentioned in the reference section. Nevertheless, at least some glimmering of the technology's power must be given here so that the its possible consequences will be obvious.

> **Nothing exists except atoms and empty space; everything else is opinion.**
>
> **Democritus**

At a basic level, everything around you is composed of atoms. Our world, all the creatures on it, the air, our bodies and our brains—all are composed of atoms. The atoms are arranged in different patterns, each pattern representing a different kind of molecule. The molecules then form together to become basic substances. A familiar example is H_2O—two hydrogen atoms and one oxygen atom combine, forming a water molecule. Everything you can see and touch can be described by these patterns, this clumping together of molecules into substance.

Drexler's vision is that we will gain control of things at the molecular level. Therefore, we will be able to build material substances to whatever precise configuration we desire. Furthermore, we will be able to do so very quickly and inexpensively.

Wouldn't some very significant scientific breakthroughs have to occur before there would be anything to get excited about?

No, the science is already done. All that's left now is engineering. Mind you, the sophistication of the required engineering is nothing to be sneered at, but use of the technology does not require any basic science breakthroughs.

> **The science of today is the technology of tomorrow.**
>
> **Edward Teller**

Drexler has repeatedly made the point that the basic science is already in place, and in fact he characterizes what he and others are doing now as "theoretical applied engineering." It is theoretical because the devices do not yet exist which will allow us to control the placement of molecules with three-dimensional precision. Progress is being made in that direction and will be discussed later. What Drexler and his cohorts are doing at this point is *assuming* that such control will be available in the future. Until precise molecular control is available, the engineering will remain theoretical.

In the meantime, those interested in nanotechnology are essentially designing the machinery, nanomachines to be built at the molecular level, that would be used in the manufacturing process. This machinery will give us the ability to produce materials with molecular precision. Though the machinery is of nanometer scale, it nevertheless is made up of familiar parts such as gears, belts, pumps, and bearings (see, for instance, Drexler, 1992, Chapters 10, 11).

Nanotechnologists are also designing computers which will operate at the molecular level. For the sake of simplicity, the design they are using for these "nanocomputers" is a mechanical one. Electronic computers, such as we are familiar with, are feasible at the nano level, but present some complications. The mechanical nanocomputers will use a logic system based on sliding rods, and will be able to communicate with nanomachines, other nanocomputers, and with macro scale computers (Drexler, 1992). Just to give you some idea of the scale involved, a mechanical nanocomputer with power equivalent to today's desktop computers would fit inside a 400 nanometer cube. Since a typical cell from the human body has a volume over a thousand times larger than that, there will plenty of room for nanocomputers and associated machinery to operate within the cell.

This size comparison gives a notion of where we are headed. Computers and machines which can fit inside a human cell could obviously be programmed to make repairs to that cell and to thus keep your body in prime condition.

Yeah, but isn't that just science fiction?

Dismissing something as science fiction is an easy and popular way to avoid thinking very hard about issues. But, is it a valid criticism? The list of technological innovations which first reached the public consciousness as science fiction is quite lengthy. To mention but a few, the list includes space travel, the use of satellites for communications, and the atomic bomb.

Of course, some things labeled as science fiction clearly *are* science fiction in the pejorative sense of the word. They are things which were improbable when written about and remain improbable. Time travel and traveling faster than the speed of light are examples of the improbable. What matters is not whether something *sounds* like science fiction, but whether there is a plausible path between the current status of the idea or technology and the future state described by the science fiction.

So, how do you decide what's plausible and what's not? Well, one easy rule of thumb is that if the concept violates any known laws of science, like traveling through time or exceeding the speed of light, it is implausible. (In using those examples I'm ignoring some wild concepts on the very edge of current thought such as worm holes, etc..)

If someone dismisses an idea, such as immortality, as science fiction, I would urge you to examine the basis of the idea. Is it implausible? If so, don't waste any time thinking about it. In this context, it is important to know that the basis of nanotechnology is not controversial and does not violate any laws of science.

If an idea is plausible, then other factors come into play. Time to fruition, for instance, represents another valid dimension for evaluating ideas. What has to happen between now and the fruition of the idea? How long is that likely to take? The idea may be plausible, and not violate any known laws of the universe, but if it's likely to take several thousand years to develop, most people, including me, are not likely to get too excited about it.

> **Time is a great teacher, but**
> **unfortunately it kills**
> **all its pupils.**
>
> **Hector Berlioz**

OK, let's go back to that business about control of things at the molecular level. Since all of this is theoretical until that's achieved, aren't you still talking about some sort of wildly unlikely scientific breakthrough?

No. There are at least two paths leading to control at the molecular level. Both are ongoing, and both are being developed by scientists and engineers in a variety of disciplines. Remember the genesis of nanotechnology. It is not some completely new discipline unrelated to anything else. It is made up of elements of already existing science and technology. As such, there are developments relevant to nanotechnology being made by people who have no particular interest in, or commitment to, nanotechnology.

One path to molecular level control is through developments in chemistry, molecular biology, and protein engineering. In each of these areas precise, molecular level changes are being manipulated and controlled (Drexler, 1992 pp. 508-511). Chemists, for instance, have built molecules which self-assemble into structures and make copies of themselves

The other general path is represented by attempts to uncover the atomic makeup of materials through sophisticated *proximal probes*, which position and maneuver sensing tips near surfaces with atomic precision. The scanning tunneling microscope and the atomic force microscope are both capable of probing at the nano level (see Drexler et al, 1991). There is a picture available which displays visible evidence of success in manipulating atoms. The picture shows the letters "IBM" and the letters are composed of 35 atoms precisely arranged by a scanning tunneling microscope. Naturally, the researchers who did the manipulation work at IBM (Eigler and Schweizer, 1990). You can see the picture by looking at the Eigler and Schweizer article or by looking at page ninety-seven of *Unbounding The Future* (Drexler et al, 1991). Because of the nature of this book, IBM wouldn't allow me to reproduce the picture here.

Other researchers have also demonstrated the ability to precisely place atoms and molecules. None of these researchers have had the kind of complete three-dimensional control needed for building molecular nanomachines, but clearly their efforts are a step along the way.

Figure 1 below shows the design for a piece of a nanomachine, a gear. Relevant engineering concerns, such as torque and friction, have been taken into account in the design of the gear.

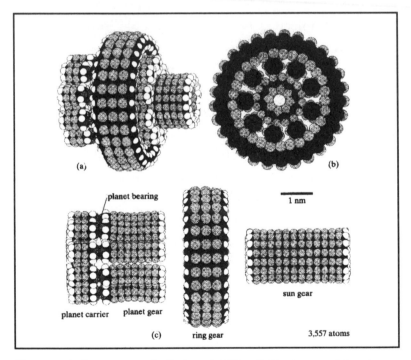

Figure 1. A planetary gear built from 3,557 individual atoms, (a) end view, (b) side view, (c) exploded view. (© 1992 John Wiley & Sons Inc. From *Nanosystems: Molecular Machinery, Manufacturing, and Computation*. All rights reserved. Reprinted with permission.)

This is design-ahead work since we do not yet have the capability to build the gear or the nanomachine it would be a part of. Once we have molecular level control, the completed design work will speed the development and fabrication of needed nanomachines. Similar design-ahead work is being carried out by Drexler and his colleagues for nanocomputers.

So you see, it's happening, it's not all just speculation. It is actual technology which is being developed as you read this book.

> The simplest schoolboy is now familiar with facts for which Archimedes would have sacrificed his life.
>
> Ernest Renan

In the fond hope you will now grant that there is some reasonable chance nanotechnology may be developed, let's go back to the main interest of this book and discuss how nanotechnology can lead to your physical immortality.

The argument is really quite straightforward. We've talked about your body as a machine. Another way to think about it, or any other material substance, is as an information pattern. The pattern of the human body can be mapped at the molecular level—no simple task, but achievable in principle through nanotechnology. Once the pattern is mapped, the information processing capability of nanocomputers and the ability of nanomachines to work at the molecular level can be harnessed together to repair and maintain the pattern, the cells, in perfect condition.

Isn't there more to the aging process than simply the wearing out of machinery in the body?

Sometimes people think of aging as a mysterious process. Ongoing research, however, is tracking down various mechanisms that lead to aging. One theory gaining in popularity attributes the effects of aging to free radicals, or destructive molecules caused by the environment and our own internal workings, which damage and destroy the body's cells. Whatever the causes of aging turn out to be, the ultimate effect is a cellular degradation.

Such cellular problems are capable of being repaired by nanomachines operating under the direction of nanocomputers. Remember, an entire nanocomputer can easily fit within one cell of your body. The nanomachines are much smaller than that, so if a cell is damaged, the damage will be reported, and the cell repaired. No aging.

If the thought of molecular mechanisms capable of making cellular repairs seems far fetched to you, consider that they already exist. Your body contains many such mechanisms provided by nature in your immune system. Nanomachines will simply improve on nature's ability to make the necessary repairs. As Drexler says, "The ill, the old, and the injured all suffer from misarranged patterns of atoms, whether misarranged by invading viruses, passing time, or swerving cars. Devices able to rearrange atoms will be able to set them right. Nanotechnology will bring a fundamental breakthrough in medicine." (Drexler, 1986, p. 99.)

Now consider this. Aging at its most basic level is the result of damaged cells. Nanotechnology will give us the ability to repair damaged cells and put them in perfect condition. Therefore nanotechnology will not only give us the ability to halt aging, but to actually *reverse the effects of aging.* No matter how old you are now, or will be when cellular repair becomes possible, we will one day have the capability to make you young again.

I'm sorry, but that sounds utterly preposterous!

It does sound strange, doesn't it? How about if I told you I could restore your automobile to factory-new condition? Suppose I had all the original specifications and the manufacturing equipment and materials to recreate any part needed. If I replace any worn parts and your car looks and drives like it just came from the showroom, would you agree that I have reversed its aging process and made it young again? With your DNA for specifications and nanotechnology to fabricate at the molecular, cellular level you too could be put in showroom condition.

In a sense you are no different than your automobile. As a biochemistry textbook states, "Living things are composed of lifeless molecules. When these molecules are isolated and examined individually, they conform to all the physical and chemical laws that describe the behavior of inanimate matter." (*Principles of Biochemistry*, 1982).

The same cellular repair strategy will serve to prevent disease. Remember that we are assuming we have a pattern for your body at the molecular level. Disease leads to change at that level and can thus be treated at that level.

But what about strange new diseases such as AIDS which have never occurred before and take years and years to unravel?

If, in fact, you have a template of your body, if you have a pattern stored showing what each cell in the body is supposed to be like, then the cause of cell damage is somewhat irrelevant. The cell simply gets repaired; the pattern is maintained at its ideal, optimal level, and you stay healthy—and immortal.

Chapter 5

Fringe Cult or
Mainstream Science?

> The scientific theory I like
> best is that the rings of Saturn
> are composed entirely of lost
> airline luggage.
>
> Mark Russell

*If this technology is really as marvelous as you describe
it, and in fact is likely to happen, why don't I already
know about it? Who's working on it? Some small band
of fanatics no one has ever heard of?*

I've mentioned Dr. Drexler's background and qualifi-
cations and that he has published three books and

numerous papers on the topic. His most recent book, *Nanosystems: Molecular Machinery, Manufacturing and Computation* (1992), provides the scientific and technological foundations for the field. A measure of its importance is that the book was honored as the computer science book of the year by the Association of American Publishers. Drexler himself received the Kilby Young Innovator Award in 1993 for his work in the field of molecular manufacturing. Of course, Drexler is by no means the only one working in the field. As mentioned earlier, nanotechnology by its nature is interdisciplinary. There are people working in a number of disciplines who would probably not identify nanotechnology as their primary professional concern, even though they are making advances which are leading to nanotechnology. Those scientists working with the scanning tunneling microscopes and those working on protein engineering provide examples.

Other evidence that nanotechnology is a growing endeavor: there is now a journal devoted to nanotechnology (see for example Drexler, 1991); there have been several conferences on the topic; there is an institute devoted to promoting the understanding of nanotechnology and its effects (The Foresight Institute); and there is an Institute for Molecular Manufacturing which funds nanotechnology research. Rice University in Houston has made a major commitment to the field and according to Rice's President, Malcolm Gillis, "Already, one-fourth of Rice's faculty in science and engineering is involved to some degree in research related to nanotechnology." The topic is also receiving attention at Harvard, MIT, and Stanford, and Princeton University is working to develop man-made molecular machines. The Beckman Institute for Advanced Science and Technology at the University of Illinois at Urbana–Champaign is organizing around three "themes" one of which is molecular and electronic nanostructures. The University of Southern California, in the Fall of 1994 established The Laboratory for Molecular Robotics.

Testimony regarding nanotechnology was given in a congressional hearing chaired by then-senator Al Gore in the fall of 1992 and met with a positive response. The hearing was about environmental concerns, and you will see how nanotechnology fits into that picture later on. Nanotechnology was also discussed in a report to the President (Science and Technology, 1993). In a recent address to the National Conference on Manufacturing Needs of U.S. Industry, the Director of the White House Office of Science and Technology Policy, Dr. Jack Gibbons, stressed the importance of nanotechnology. He said in part, "This new technology could fuel a powerful economic engine providing new sources of jobs and wealth and technology spillover." (Foresight Update, 1995, p.14) Drexler has given many lectures on nanotechnology to a variety of scientific audiences and reports that the concept has never been successfully refuted. "Molecular nanotechnology falls entirely within the realm of the possible." (Drexler, Peterson and Pergamit, 1991)

Here's another little item that might help you believe that nanotechnology is a real possibility. If I were to ask you what country in the world is best at taking other people's basic technological ideas and turning them into very marketable products, you'd probably have no trouble coming up with Japan as the answer. It is of more than passing interest, then, to note that the Ministry of International Trade and Industry in Japan has recently funded a $200 million, ten-year nanotechnology project. Other Japanese agencies are also working in nanotechnology research and development with approximately another $300 million in funding.

Now, in the grand scheme of things, $500 million is not a gigantic commitment. It's not chopped liver, either. Of course, you may know that Japan funded another project over a ten-year period with the purpose of developing fifth generation computer technology, computers which would think like humans and respond to interactive voice commands. After much money and effort, the project was abandoned. So, the mere fact that the Japanese have devoted money to something does not mean that they will necessarily develop it. Given the relative economic track records of our respective countries in recent years, however, ignoring the topic would not seem to be in our best self interest.

Nor are the Japanese the only ones to have an interest. A Nanotechnology Facility has been proposed in Australia, and Switzerland has budgeted over $17 million for nanoscience research over the next five years.

> The race not always to the
> swift nor the battle
> to the strong — but that's
> the way to bet it.
>
> Damon Runyon

I'm not sure immortality is such a good idea. Maybe all
these researchers or their governments will come to the
same conclusion, and the research area will be dropped.

Once something has been shown to be both feasible
and desirable, the chances are very good it will be developed somewhere by someone. The history of mankind is
full of multiple, simultaneous inventions. Calculus was
invented (or at least reported on) nearly simultaneously
and independently by Leibniz and Newton in the 17th
century. Many early varieties of automobile were developed independently of one another. Several others were
working on airplanes when the Wright brothers first
flew. The list of synchronous discoveries is quite lengthy,
and the principle quite obvious. If nanotechnology
should fall out of favor with one group of researchers or
one country, it is highly unlikely that that will be the
end of it.

> **What is possible for technology to do, technology will have done...regardless, regardless of anything.**
>
> **Archibald MacLeish**

Of course, as an old professor of mine liked to say, rare events happen...rarely. Catastrophic events could intervene. A large astroid could strike the earth, or a virulent unstoppable plague could quickly sweep the planet. Either of these events would surely derail any new technological advances, in addition to their other more horrific effects. Barring any such catastrophes, however, mankind seems bent on improving its control over the material world—and nanotechnology will represent the ultimate in that control. Man's imagination provides many barriers, nature few.

Well, what about cost? Cellular repair nanotechnology sounds like something only rich people will be able to afford.

Initially that may be true, but costs for high technology have a way of going down rapidly. Nanotechnology costs, for reasons to be explained later having to do with production costs, most likely will plummet even more steeply than earlier technologies. *Cryonics* (1993, p.51) presents an interesting analogy, involving the semiconductor liquid crystal display (LCD) wristwatch. Not too many years ago you could spend several hundred dollars on a jeweled, Swiss movement, state-of-the-art wristwatch that kept pretty fair time. Today you can buy an electronic, LCD wristwatch which keeps excellent time for $3. In 1965 no amount of money would have purchased such a precise, light, dependable watch. The start-up costs of developing cellular repair nanotechnology will no doubt be huge, but the patient man-in-the-street will eventually be easily able to afford its cost.

> Why do we call our generous
> ideas illusions, and the
> mean ones truth?
>
> **Edith Wharton**

Chapter 6

Timing is Everything:
Will You Make It?

> Time is that which man is
> always trying to kill, but
> which ends in killing him.
>
> Herbert Spencer

OK, for the sake of argument, suppose I admit that nanotechnology is going to happen. It's not likely to happen in my lifetime, is it?

That, of course, is a question of prime interest in a book which claims to be telling you how you can

become immortal. We've laid out a scenario of technological advance which will make immortality practical.
The question is, will you be around when the scenario
reaches fruition? There are several parts to the answer.

A key part of the answer concerns the question of
how long it will take before nanotechnology moves from
the realm of *theoretical* applied engineering and becomes
simply *applied* engineering. So, let's try to answer that
question first.

The nanotechnology literature contains implementa-
tion estimates ranging from ten years to one hundred
years. No one expresses any confidence in their ability, or
the ability of anyone else, to come up with a precise date.
There are just too many unknowns. But the disagreement
is not about "if," just about "when." Once the technology
becomes feasible, advances may be incredibly rapid.

Computer technology provides an interesting, analo-
gous example. Fifteen years ago I managed a computer
installation which cost over one hundred thousand dollars, filled a room, and took four people to operate. It
had less than a tenth of the capacity of the $2,000 laptop
computer I am using to write this book. And my computer itself is two generations out of date—two generations which took four years.

Clearly, with the kinds of enormous changes that can
take place rapidly, technology is a difficult area in which
to make predictions regarding timing. Drexler quotes a
colleague of his as making an optimistic prediction that it
will take thirty years before nanotechnology is developed.

That same colleague's pessimistic prediction is ten years. The pessimism relates to the enormous social changes that will accompany a mature nanotechnology. (see Drexler, 1986 and also Chapter 9) More recently Drexler has given two different "conservative" estimates. "If you are considering the benefits of nanotechnology, it is conservative to plan on 20 years. If you are concerned about competitors getting it first, it is conservative to plan on 10 years." (Foresight Update, 1995, p.20)

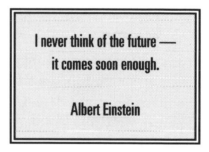

Concerning the speed at which nanotechnology will transform our world, whenever the transformation starts, Drexler draws interesting arguments from history (1988). Examples of abrupt changes in our technological capabilities include communications going from the speed of horses to near the speed of light with the invention of the telegraph, and the over a million-fold increase in the amount of energy we could release from a chunk of matter with the invention of the atomic bomb. Chances are the nanotechnology transformation will also be very rapid. Nanotechnology will allow for the introduction of large quantities of both familiar and novel products, inexpensively produced, in very short time periods. That abundance, and the fact that the production methods will be unlike any others we have known, will be the driving forces behind rapid changes.

So, back to the original question about whether nanotechnology will be developed during the lifetime of someone reading this book. Clearly, it will be in your favor if you are young, are in good health, have a healthy lifestyle, and have inherited good longevity genes. Race car driving and bungee jumping most likely will work against you. The question, however, does not have a firm answer. One factor complicating the issue is that all the different applications of nanotechnology will not be simultaneously developed. One of the most involved applications will be cellular repair, so it is not likely to be among the first developments.

One could argue that as the average life span continues to lengthen, the older you get the better your chances for living even longer.

Every day above ground is a good one.

Bumper Sticker

There is a flaw in that argument, however, because most of the increase in life expectancy is a result of more people living past infancy, rather than a result of people getting older and older. People don't tend to reach any older age now than they did years ago. More people are reaching those older ages, and chances are they will be healthier getting there, but so far we haven't licked the problem of the machine wearing out at some point. Current thinking is that the human life span is limited to 110 to 120 years.

Drexler presents an interesting sort of bootstrap argument in *Engines of Creation*. The basic notion is that research on preventing death is an ongoing proposition. His argument is that as time goes on we will eventually solve each of the problems that now lead to death. That gradual progress, then, may lengthen the life span of those now alive so that they are able to reach a time when nanotechnology will make cell repair available. The scenario would be that just as you are about to expire from heart disease, a new technique solves that problem...allowing you to live long enough that a cure is found for the liver cancer you next develop...which allows you to live until...and so on until cellular repair nanotechnology is developed.

Still and all, things could be said to look a little chancy as to whether you and I will make it through until that time. There is another step you can take, however, to significantly improve your odds of reaching the era of cellular repair nanotechnology. That step is to enter a state of biostasis. The latter part of this book will address that topic.

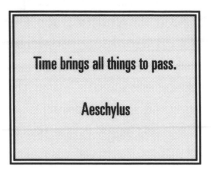

Time brings all things to pass.

Aeschylus

For now, let's assume for the sake of argument that you can reach the time when near immortality is within your grasp. Let's move on to some other possible objections you might have. What has gone before has been an attempt to persuade you that someday immortality may be a viable option, a real possibility. Are you convinced?

Chapter 7

Bodies, Bodies Everywhere

> We have been God-like in our planned breeding of our domestic plants and animals, but rabbit-like in our unplanned breeding of ourselves.
>
> Arnold Toynbee

OK, once again for the sake of argument I'll grant the possibility of immortality, but how about all the other horrific problems the world suffers from now. Wouldn't immortality just make them much worse—for instance, what about overpopulation?

Well now, it's probably time to drop the other shoe. What I've focused on so far, because it is the main topic, is the prospect of you becoming immortal. The other shoe has to do with all the other mind-boggling aspects of a mature nanotechnology.

One of the most profound implications of nanotechnology has to do with the cost of manufactured goods. Two of the basic and significant costs of manufactured goods are the cost of the raw materials and the labor costs associated with turning those raw materials into finished products. Using nanotechnology, a very high percentage of the labor will be provided by self-replicating nanomachines, and the raw materials needed will be very inexpensive bulk chemicals in such forms as gasoline, methanol, ammonia and hydrogen.

One of the key concepts of nanotechnology is that of assemblers. These will be the nanomachines which, in concert, will actually produce the goods we need. One of the things they can be programmed to do is to replicate themselves. Assuming sufficient materials to work with, one replicator, needing a 15-minute cycle to copy itself, can produce 68 billion copies of itself in a ten-hour period (Drexler, 1986, pp.57-58). Sound implausible? Bacteria can replicate at that rate, and conservative calculations suggest that nanomachines will be able to also.

One will simply feed in a slurry of basic building block materials containing the atoms needed to build the desired end product. Sometime later, on the order of an hour or less for many objects, the finished product will be available.

Aren't you just describing magic?

> **Any sufficiently advanced technology is indistinguishable from magic.**
>
> **Arthur C. Clarke**

Sounds like magic—but it's just technology. One of the ways to try to capture the power of nanotechnology is to think of a nanocomputer containing all of the necessary information to build a sophisticated finished product, say a microwave oven, as a seed. The nanocomputer is placed in an environment containing self-replicating assembler devices and the necessary feedstock to produce the object. And away the system goes, assembling the object atom by atom, molecule by molecule, until the seed has grown into whatever was imprinted in its programming, a mighty oak—or the latest in microwaves. Naturally occurring seeds perform these wonders every day; man-made nanoseeds will also.

Nanotechnology will bring about an era of material abundance like none ever before seen. All of the normal manufacturing cost factors, such as labor, raw materials, design and energy, will be significantly less when goods are produced by molecular manufacturing and design can be carried out by artificial intelligences. Every home and business will be able to afford a molecular manufacturing unit capable of building a wide variety of products using very inexpensive chemical feedstock for material. And, the unit will produce rather than consume energy. Sound too good to be true? So might many things such as antibiotics, worldwide communications, and computers have sounded to our ancestors of not very long ago.

Overpopulation manifests itself as a host of problems. In order to think about the effects of nanotechnology and immortality, one must break down the problem of overpopulation into its component parts. Nanotechnology can eliminate some problems such as disease and illness, and alleviate others such as food shortages, overcrowding, and lack of material goods. We should be clear from the start, however, that no technology can overcome the effects of unlimited geometric population growth.

What is "geometric" growth?

In this case, it refers to the capability of a population to grow by some ratio, such as doubling, or tripling or quadrupling, in a fixed period of time. Any population growing at a geometric rate, as the human race is capable of doing, can outstrip natural resources of any magnitude, including those of a whole galaxy. How fast that happens depends on how quickly the population reproduces. Overpopulation is a problem for our race regardless of whether humans have a short or long life span.

As mentioned earlier in reference to self-replicating nanoassemblers, if the reproduction time necessary to double the population is fifteen minutes, a sweet two-some can grow to an astonishing sixty-eight billion-some in just ten hours. Humans, operating at maximum efficiency, would take close to ten years rather than fifteen minutes to double the population size, but the eventual outcome can be just as awesome. So, some constraints on population growth obviously will occur no matter how powerful the technology. It is comforting to note in this respect that there is some evidence that material abundance and population growth are inversely related (Rubenstein, 1994). That is, as the standard of living increases the rate of population growth goes down. In most of the industrialized nations fertility rates are below the replacement level. If that trend holds in the future, overpopulation may not be as much of a problem as we currently fear.

The faces of overpopulation we are most familiar with from our television screens are those of malnutrition and disease. In a society of immortal beings there will be no disease. Disease implies change in the template of your body pattern, and that template is exactly what will be maintained through nanotechnology—therefore, no disease.

Food supply is dependent upon many things, such as arable land, weather patterns, distribution systems, and water supply. Nanotechnology will make fundamental changes in many of these areas and will make possible the production of finished food products from basic raw materials. But, again, keep in mind that unlimited population growth can exceed any production system no matter how sophisticated and technologically advanced it may be. Nanotechnology will help support a much larger population than we can currently feed, but we as a race will still have to exercise some form of control over our population growth.

Let's suppose you're right and we'll keep the population sufficiently in check that we can feed people and that they will have material comforts. Still, you're talking about adding millions and millions and billions of people to the population. Pretty soon there won't even be room to stand. We'll be stacked on top of each other like logs.

Yes, but there's space in space. Understanding the implications of nanotechnology requires making a paradigm shift. It's a new ball game with a new set of rules, and a lot of the old rules don't apply. With the *caveat* mentioned earlier that no technology can cope with geometric population growth, nanotechnology will open vast and practically unlimited habitable living space to the human race.

Basically nanotechnology will make everything less expensive including, in particular, solar energy, transportation, and material goods. Consequently, currently uninhabitable areas of the Earth's surface will become inhabitable. Efficient, inexpensive solar power, employing virtually indestructible nano-assembled materials, for instance, should provide all the energy anyone needs to live anywhere they want.

Our satellite system provides essentially instantaneous global communications. According to popular reports, we are not many years removed from using the equivalent of a cellular phone to communicate from any spot on the Earth's surface to another.

With less expensive, less polluting transportation (to be discussed later), transportation which does not eat so voraciously into the earth's limited resources, shipping ourselves and our goods around will be easier and have much less impact on the environment than present day practices.

The combined capabilities of nanotechnology will make it possible and attractive to live not only on land, but also on the sea, under the sea, and underground. All in all, the Earth will be able to support many more people in comfort than it can currently.

The real space bonanza, however, occurs in space. With nanomachines to assemble whatever physical products we want, cheap reliable space flight will become available. Drexler, in *Engines of Creation*, presents an interesting scenario of a rocket engine being created using nanotechnology. The engine, conventional in overall design but superior in many ways (it is essentially constructed of diamond), is grown from a nano "seed" with virtually no human intervention in less than a day—and it is very inexpensive.

With cheap space transportation, an asteroid system full of building materials and with nanoassemblers to build whatever we want, there is no reason why large, luxurious habitats cannot be built in space, both in near-Earth orbit and at other places in the solar system. These habitats, rotated to provide gravity, would contain cities, lakes, rivers, and mountains in a plentitude of different landscapes and living arrangements. You can read descriptions of such habitats and their possibilities in *The High Frontier: Human Colonies in Space* by Gerard K. O'Neill (1976). The space frontier will provide not only living room, but room for new ideas, new ways of doing things. If a society of immortals on Earth appears too hidebound, there will be other places to go to try new ideas, new ways of living.

Expansion to other star systems is also a possibility, although presumably not one which would ever relieve much of the population pressure on Earth because of the time it would take to reach other systems. We have already sent the Voyager I and II spacecraft to the stars . There is no reason in principle why we could not send humans on board such spacecraft. Granted it would be a long flight to even the nearest star systems at sub-light speeds, but with immortality and the mastering of biostasis there is no reason why humans could not make such a journey. This possibility will be discussed further in a later chapter.

To sum up, nanotechnology will make possible immortality, and immortality could obviously worsen our overpopulation problems. Nanotechnology will also provide the means, however, to solve those very same problems. It will do so by providing us with abundant material goods, perfect health, and the ability to vastly expand our habitat.

> **The only limit to our realization of tomorrow will be our doubts of today.**
>
> **Franklin D. Roosevelt**

CHAPTER 8

Fooling with Mother Nature: Pollution and the Natural Order

> I shot an arrow into the
> sky...and it stuck.
>
> Graffito in Los Angeles

Travel to the stars! Let's talk about something a little closer to home. Even if we somehow find the space we'll need for all these additional people you're talking about, what about the environment? We already have it trashed out pretty badly and now you're wanting to add billions of more people to the problem.

The environment problem can be broken into two parts. The first part is comprised of damage we have done to the environment so far and the further damage we will do before nanotechnology becomes available. The second part concerns the impact a society of immortals, working with nanotechnology, will have on the environment. Although it may seem counter-intuitive, let's deal with the future first.

We currently pollute our world in a variety of ways including the noxious, hazardous by-products of the manufacturing process; the by-products of generating power (whether it be power to heat and cool our homes and run our machines, or the power needed for transportation in the form of automobiles, buses, trucks, trains, and airplanes); and the sewage and other waste materials of the human condition. Nanotechnology provides solutions to all these pollution problems.

A manufacturing process controlled at the atomic level will generate precious few noxious by-products. Molecular manufacturing will make possible vast efficiencies in current solar energy technology and battery longevity and performance. Drexler *et al.*(1991) speculate on repaving our highways with extremely efficient solar panels which will be both inexpensive and nearly indestructible. The only potentially harmful by-product so far identified for molecular manufacturing is a certain amount of waste heat.

One part of the current manufacturing process which produces both material and visual pollution is the mining industry. Billions of nanomachines can be programmed to extract any material we want from the ground or the sea and leave no visible trace or by-products. They will also make possible very efficient recycling of discarded materials by breaking them down into their constituent molecules and then building anew. Recycling based on nanotechnology will work just as well for organic (sewage, waste water, etc.) as for inorganic materials.

Transportation is another major source of pollution in today's world. Nanotechnology will help us develop practical electric cars by providing extremely strong, durable and lightweight materials. It will also aid in the production of very efficient batteries to power those cars. Cheap digging machines, cheaply manufactured passenger cars, cheap super-computers (to direct traffic), cheap superconductor materials, and solar energy will all combine to make possible a vast network of linked, underground transportation. Transportation through the tunnels on magnetically levitated capsules riding over superconducting tracks could be fast, comfortable, user-friendly and minimally polluting.

Well, OK, that's fine for the future, assuming it's all true, but what about the mess we're in right now? Adding more people, even with molecular manufacturing, can only make things worse.

Nanotechnology can rid us of some of the more embarrassing monuments to our past excesses. Nanomachines could be turned loose on toxic waste dumps to disassemble the harmful substances at the molecular level and render them harmless. Polluted rivers and bodies of water could be cleared in the same fashion. Drexler (Drexler *et al.,* 1991) has even proposed an ingenious scheme for using nanotechnology to cleanse the stratosphere of ozone destroying pollutants. In short, nanotechnology will help us heal and cleanse our troubled planet, and provide the means to keep it nearly pristine.

People worry rightly about the carrying capacity of the Earth and about the damage we are doing to other life forms on the planet. Nanotechnology will significantly increase the planet's carrying capacity by reducing the polluting effects of our industries and by vastly increasing our ability to provide the material goods needed to support life. It will also provide a means to repair the damaged habitats of other animal species.

The situation we're in right now is that there are only two ways to increase the level of material comfort for the world's population. One way is to crank up production and further stress, or even destroy, the planet's capability to maintain itself. The other way is to give everyone a bigger piece of the pie by reducing the number of pie seekers—the population. Nanotechnology gives us a third option. Since it will increase the carrying capacity of the planet, we will be able to upgrade the quality of life for everyone without damaging the planet.

As mentioned previously, of course, we could out-breed even the capabilities of nanotechnology. The technology doesn't make the problem of overpopulation go away, but it does give us a way to recover from our current problems. The essence of the argument is that a society of immortals, in conjunction with nanotechnology, need not add to overpopulation and pollution problems. Such a society can alleviate our current problems and lead to a saner, richer, less crowded, much less polluted world.

However, the fact that nanotechnology may eventually help with our environmental problems should not deter current efforts to improve. We have to live in the here-and-now, and here and now the environment needs help. We should be working simultaneously towards a cleaner environment *and* the development of nanotechnology.

It seems to me that immortality is against nature, against the natural order of things.

That's true in the sense that the natural thing for an organism to do is die (although some trees, for instance, take a lot longer to do the natural thing than a human). But from that point of view we went off the tracks a long time ago. Any intervention to prevent a person from dying can be considered unnatural. I believe that most people would argue that modern medicine is a positive thing even though it might be unnatural (and expensive).

Modern medicine has among its goals improving the quality of life and extending it as much as possible. These goals will be greatly furthered by nanotechnology. If you feel the life extending qualities of nanotechnology are unnatural, do you feel the same way about a person taking an antibiotic to cure pneumonia or insulin to control diabetes? The difference is only one of magnitude. Nanotechnology and antibiotics are both unnatural.

> The one consistently natural thing is to try by intelligence and imagination to improve on nature.
>
> Brigid Brophy

Of course, one can also argue that man is a creature of nature and that anything man creates is, *ipso facto*, natural. I prefer to think that the mechanisms nature provided for our health and longevity can be improved upon, and any improvements we make are cause for celebration and a tribute to our ingenuity.

Given all the capabilities you've talked about and given the changes we'll be able to make in our bodies, are you sure the human race will still be "human"?

It is true that nanotechnology will enable humans to make some startling changes. The obvious ones, the ones we've talked about the most, are freedom from the effects of disease and aging. These changes will lead to immortality. You could think of these, however, as not altering the essential nature of human beings, merely clearing up some defects. For now, though, let's hold the picture right there. There are many other changes possible, and we'll talk about some of them a little later, but even with just the changes mentioned it is possible to say that humans will be dramatically transformed.

For one thing of course, people will no longer be able to say, "Life is too short for...." Though it sounds like a joke, there is actually a serious point to be made here— that the basic framework against which almost all human thought takes place will change. In that framework, death is a certain and blighting shadow on our future. This fact surely colors our thoughts in a multitude of ways, some obvious and others operating at the unconscious level.

So, would beings who don't have near, imminent death always looming in the future be human or something else? I would argue that they are still humans, just humans relieved of a heavy psychological burden under which mankind has labored throughout its entire history. Take yourself, for instance. Suppose you were suddenly told that you no longer had to worry about dying, that you were going to live forever. Do you think you would become inhuman? I think not.

> **I am a man. Nothing human is**
> **alien to me.**
>
> **The poet Terence**

Now, let's unfreeze the picture and talk about other kinds of changes that might take place. For instance, let's talk about your physical appearance. If nanoseeds can build rocket engines and other sophisticated devices and can make repairs to your body at the cellular level, they can surely make a new you. Do you want to be taller? shorter? thinner? No problem. Do you want to be handsomer or prettier? How about the color of your skin? The shape of your eyes? Want to look Asian? White? Black?

In an age when one's looks are a matter of choice, handsome and pretty may no longer have much true meaning or impact, at least from the point of view of social desirability. We may instead be dealing in degrees of eccentricity. Do you want to look unusual? What effect will these kinds of changes have on the attraction between the sexes, when desirable sexual characteristics such as size of breasts and hips, musculature, height and facial features are a matter of choice? How will you decide whom to mate with?

For that matter, what sex do you want to be? With cellular level control, and the right road map, changing from male to female or vice versa should be possible. And remember that these are not idle questions that some stranger in the future may be dealing with, but questions relevant to you if you should choose to live in that future. The choice is yours.

How about something more exotic. Want to fly? What if we make your bones hollow and grow some wings for you so that you can soar with eagles. Are you still human when you're soaring? I think so, others might not.

If you can change your physical appearance, how about your information processing capability, your ability to compute? Since nanocomputers will fit inside a human cell, clearly we can add computers to the cells of your brain, make the necessary linkages, and vastly increase your ability to retain and process information. Are you still a human when those changes have been made? Maybe you're not *homo sapiens* anymore, but rather *homo computeris*.

There are many variations of this line of thought that could be explored and played out. The essential point is that we will have the ability to change ourselves in dramatic and heretofore impossible ways. These capabilities may in fact change the human experience to a sufficient degree that we will no longer be the *homo sapiens* we have been for the last million years or so. The question of who will be in charge of the changes is an important one. Who will decide what humans are supposed to be like? This is only one of the many fundamental issues which will have to be dealt with as nanotechnology matures.

So, what does one do with this kind of information? Is it cause for not developing nanotechnology and therefore not reaping all the other benefits nanotechnology will bring? I've argued that stopping the development of a technology once it has begun seems to be impossible. If that's true, we don't have any choice.

One way to view what will take place is to observe that our species has been changing over millennia through natural evolution. At this point we are taking evolution into our own hands, and not in any subtle way either. If you could have asked Lucy, the australopithicene found years ago by Dr. Richard Leakey, whether she wanted to evolve into *homo sapiens*, she might have said thanks, but no. She didn't have a choice and we probably don't either. The best we can do, as in other areas of our lives which will be transformed by nanotechnology, is to anticipate that the changes will be occurring and try to prepare ourselves, prepare our path, as best we can.

Some of the kinds of changes discussed above probably seem bizarre or even distasteful. That does not mean they are not possible. It is important to make a distinction between what man wants or finds acceptable and what nature allows. The laws of the universe exist independent of human desires. If it can be done, it probably will be done.

We are in collision with tomorrow. Future shock has arrived.

Alvin Toffler

CHAPTER 9

Fooling with Institutions: Insurance, Medicine and the Economy

> All progress is initiated by challenging current conceptions, and executed by supplanting existing institutions,
>
> Bernard Shaw

It seems to me that any technology as powerful as the one you're talking about—which can manufacture nearly anything cheaply, clean up the environment, make us immortal—is going to lead to major, major changes in the way we live. Won't that cause problems?

The age of nanotechnology will be vastly different from the world we live in now, and moving from our current society to a society with nanotechnology at its center will undoubtedly cause severe disruptions along the way. Let's talk about the scope of the change for a moment. Human progress over the years is generally broken into four time periods or ages: the hunting/gathering age, agricultural age, industrial age, and our current information age. The underlying differences in how people provided themselves with the essentials of life during each of these ages necessarily led to fundamental, qualitative differences in the very texture of their day-to-day existence. To take an extreme example, depending for your supper on your most recent success in killing an animal or finding edible roots is quite different from popping your TV dinner in the microwave. Both give you necessary sustenance, but they require wildly diverse sets of skills and support mechanisms to bring about.

The transition from one period to the next causes disruptions in many societal mechanisms. For instance, some professions become nearly obsolete (buggy whip maker, coal stoker, pony express rider), and new ones spring up (automobile mechanic, computer programmer). Moving from the information age to the nanotechnology age will bring about as much change and disruption as did the move from an agricultural society to an industrial one, or the move from an industrial society to the information society we currently live in. The scope of these changes will be staggering and in general beyond the purview of this book. It does make sense, however, to talk a little bit about the changes which will take place. Such a discussion will give you some inkling of the kinds of upheaval that are likely to occur in our future and our children's future.

Though precise predictions of social and technological changes are very difficult to make, it is not as difficult to paint in a few broad brush strokes. A number of our major institutions will change dramatically or change so much they will no longer be recognizable. To take one example, what role would there be for people selling life insurance in a world where true death is a very rare event? What happens to health insurance when aging and disease have been conquered? Clearly from the point of view of these kinds of organizations, and their stockholders, the consequences of nanotechnology will be very negative.

From the point of view of mankind as a whole, many would contend that the disappearance of life insurance sales agents is not a strong argument against immortality. Even the stockholders in such companies, if not too much of their assets are tied up in them, might prefer to trade off the value of their stock for a chance at personal immortality. Of course, none of these things will happen overnight, so there will be plenty of time for those with foresight to adapt. The idea will be to get out of buggy-whip manufacturing well before the world is covered with automobiles. Upheaval? Yes. Bad? Only for some, and only for a limited period of time.

The conquering of age and disease will cause similar large scale problems for the medical complex. What tools or treatment are needed when everyone has nanomachines inside them capable of repairing body cells which become aberrant? There will still be a need for basic medical research and for facilities to treat those whose repair needs are extensive and time consuming. But meeting those needs will require nothing like the large scale all-purpose medical complex we have now— and will lead to nothing like the expenses currently associated with such services.

When people are no longer dying to get into the cemetery, what will happen to the funeral industry? If any industry will be directly affected by nanotechnology, it will be that one. There will be a significant lack of business for everyone from undertakers to grave diggers.

The effects of nanotechnology will not be limited to institutions affected by human health and longevity. Nanotechnology will represent a basic change in the way material goods are produced and that change means many other institutions and industries will be disrupted. For instance, what will be the function of utility companies in an era when nanotechnology has made solar energy incredibly cheap to produce? Using some basic figures provided by Drexler, Merkle estimates that a one square meter solar cell can be produced by molecular manufacturing for a cost of less than a penny. Electric power, which now costs about ten cents per kilowatt hour, will cost about three <u>millicents</u> per kilowatt hour in the era of nanotechnology (Merkle, 1994). Imagine the ripple effect produced by having access to power which is several thousand times cheaper than that available today.

> **The art of progress is to preserve order amid change, and to preserve change amid order.**
>
> **A. N. Whitehead**

Of course, when we discuss any particular industry or institution, such as the medical profession, insurance, or utilities, we should realize that not only will those industries be affected, but all the others that are dependent upon them also. Utilities, for instance, use wire for transmitting their power. The wire has to be purchased from a manufacturer. If the utility company has a drastically changed business, the need for wire will disappear, and the manufacturers of wire will be caught in same upheaval as everyone else. This dependency effect will be multiplied many times.

If you would like a more mundane example, consider the plight of mom-and-pop dry cleaning shops when "smart" clothing becomes available. Smart clothing will be manufactured by nanomachines and will also contain nanomachines (remember they are much smaller than a human body cell) with the assignment of removing any foreign material which becomes attached to the garment, such as dirt. What need for dry cleaners then?

One can imagine the scheming and maneuvering likely to go on in the stock market as nanotechnology becomes feasible and everyone tries to figure out which stocks will go up and which will go down. In that context, companies holding the basic patents in nanotechnology will be very good bets. Those who are investment minded and think in the long term might begin to look at technologies and companies out of which nanotechnology is likely to develop, such as biotechnological research companies and companies manufacturing the kinds of tools which might be used to manipulate matter at the atomic level, e.g., the atomic force microscope, the scanning tunneling microscope.

To mention one more topic, consider precious gems. Gems such as diamonds have fired man's imagination, artistic endeavors and greed for millennia. Many people display their wealth in the form of diamonds and other precious gems they own, primarily, of course, as jewelry. Remember that nanotechnology with its control at the molecular level allows one to build virtually any material from very inexpensive feedstock materials. Remember also Drexler's example of a spacecraft engine essentially made of diamond. Now think about the holders of precious gems such as diamonds when those materials can be made in inexpensive abundance by the philosopher's stone of nanotechnology. You should be clear that we are talking not about materials "like" diamond but material indistinguishable from diamond at the atomic level.

The same argument can be extended to any other natural material, such as those extracted from the earth. So now we have another industry, the mining industry, which will undergo major change because of nanotechnology. The examples are nearly endless, but the point is the same—nanotechnology will represent a fundamental change in the way the world operates. Many societal institutions and mechanisms will be changed beyond recognition. Undoubtedly, many people will feel the disruptive force of nanotechnology as their buggy whip plants go out of business or move into a different business altogether.

To combat these disruptions, Drexler and others urge that the public begin setting up mechanisms to deal with the change and begin debating and deciding what kind of society we want to have and what sorts of new institutions and new ways of conducting our affairs will help us handle the transition. Right at the moment not very many people have heard that message, so the debate is not yet under way.

Obviously, change of the magnitude being discussed will be harmful to many. Even if it were possible to delay the change by delaying nanotechnology, one could easily argue that we shouldn't do that because of all the advantages nanotechnology will bring. But, as we have seen in the discussion about multiple simultaneous inventions, trying to stop such a technological change once the seeds have been sown, once we have reached the stage of progress where this technology is possible, is likely to be impossible anyway. Our best bet then is not to say that nanotechnology will cause too many problems, that immortality is an uncomfortable thought, that we shouldn't develop nanotechnology. Our best bet is to prepare for the change as quickly and as ably as we can.

CHAPTER 10

Sacrilege, Boredom and Your 500th Wedding Anniversary

> There is so little difference between husbands you might as well keep the first.
>
> Adela Rogers St. Johns

How about religion? This must surely be against most people's religious beliefs.

By and large, religions don't have any injunctions against life extension techniques. Christian Scientists and those religions, such as the Jehovah's Witnesses, which prohibit blood transfusions, would be exceptions. Using nanomachines to effect cellular repairs is simply another form of life preservation and extension. To those who believe in God, a very extended mortal lifetime here on Earth, or in space, would still take place in the blink of God's eye. All other factors would remain constant, except for having more time to find either God or occasions to sin.

George P. Smith, in *Medical-Legal Aspects of Cryonics: Prospects For Immortality* (1983) cites various sources as showing no conflict between religious teachings and attempts to markedly lengthen life span. If you have an immortal soul, there is no reason to suspect it will go anywhere or change in any way while your body lives on for an extended period of time.

> Everybody wants to get to heaven
> but nobody wants to die.
>
> Joe Louis

Well, it's at least unseemly if nothing else. What about all the poor, starving people in the world today? Isn't it kind of selfish to be thinking about making yourself immortal when there are so many people who can't even lead a decent life right now?

Obviously it will be viewed that way by some, but what's the reality of the situation? What effect can you have now on those poor, miserable people? On one hand you could argue that the time, money and energy you might spend on pursuing immortality for yourself could be devoted to helping the world's poor, but would it really change anything in the long run? On the other hand, your interest in immortality, and nanotechnology as a way of achieving it, may shorten, in however small a way, the time between now and when nanotechnology becomes available. If so, you will in fact have done a great deal because nanotechnology offers a permanent solution for many of the world's ills including poverty.

Say it was possible, say I did it. What in the world would I do with all that time?

Millions long for immortality who do not know what to do with themselves on a rainy Sunday afternoon.

Susan Ertz

Well, the possibilities seem endless to me. The topic of what to do with your time breaks rather naturally into two categories, work time and leisure time. Let's talk about work first.

Very few people these days leave school, start a job in a particular field, and stay with that job the rest of their working life (Mergenhagen, 1991). Career change has become the norm. There are probably several reasons for this including an increase in the number of productive years a person has available. The time people spend in a career has doubled since the turn of the century. Also, relatively rapid changes in the job market make jobs obsolete or at least overpopulated and contribute to career changes. In addition, most people are relatively well informed about other areas of endeavor, and with the rise of two-income families it is easier for a person to accept a decrease in income while they break into a new career.

There's no reason to expect things to be any different in a society of immortals. So, instead of having two or three or four careers in your lifetime, you might have a hundred or three hundred or a thousand. Keep in mind all the new frontiers inexpensive access to space will open. These new frontiers will in turn open careers we've not even dreamed of—how about a career as a low gravity landscape artist, for instance, or a job designing high fashion nanoclothing seeds?

> "What'll we do with ourselves this afternoon?" cried Daisy, "and the day after that, and the next thirty years?"
>
> F. Scott Fitzgerald

The question of leisure time bears some similarity to the work question. Research has shown that people spend roughly equal proportions of their leisure time watching television, engaging in some sort of activity, and socializing (Roberts, 1978). Most people have several hobby-type activities which they engage in over the course of their lifetime. The number and mix of them may change, but it is a fairly small number. In the time available it's hard to learn how to play a good game of chess, crochet well, collect stamps, play tennis, and watch sixty hours of television a week. For some, the activities are more sedentary, such as learning how to be a world champion channel surfer, and for others they are more active and sports related.

In any case, the number of hobby possibilities open to a person are relatively few. In an immortal society, on the other hand, one would have time to learn to do anything one wanted. Take up the piano for thirty years and learn to play it as well as you can. Then move on to astronomy or gardening or whatever suits your fancy.

How about nurturing your artistic talents? Sure, you have some. You just haven't discovered what they are yet. As Drexler observes, "To the creation of symphony and song, paintings and worlds, software, theorems, films, and delights yet unimagined, there seems no end. New technologies will nurture new arts, and new arts will bring new standards." (Drexler, 1986, p.166).

If such Earthbound pursuits seem too tame for you, join an exploration party (consisting of an ever-spreading number of clones) seeking to map the galaxy or help move stellar matter and black holes around. Both of these ideas have been proposed by H. Keith Henson in an article entitled "What To Do With a Million Years" (1993). He suggests that the galactic explorers could meet for a giant Party At The End Of The Galaxy, once their task is completed.

The difference between thinking about multiple hobbies and a complete mapping of the galaxy is a rather fundamental one. Multiple hobbies might serve to keep one happily occupied for hundreds of years. Mapping the galaxy and moving stellar material could take millions of years. For people used to thinking in decades, hundreds is a stretch, and millions are basically incomprehensible. This is clearly an area where one step at a time makes the most sense. Let's worry about that rainy afternoon first, and what to do about next week when we get there.

No matter what time scale we think about, however, it is probable that you would be bored some percentage of the time. It's not likely to be any greater a percentage of your time than it is now, though. So, if you are bored ten days out of a thousand now, you'd probably be bored ten days out of a thousand as an immortal. There would just be more of those thousand-day periods for you to enjoy.

In fact, an immortal may not be much worried about what to do with his or her time in the first place. Implicit in the worry is the notion that one has a limited number of days in which to do anything, and it's worrisome to think that you might not enjoy some of those precious few as much as you'd like. If, on the other hand, the supply of days seems endless, then what happens on any particular one is relatively less important. In any case, which problem would you rather have to deal with—making sure you don't regret the few years you have now? Or how to spend eternity?

OK, so maybe there'll be lots to do and I won't be any more bored than I am now. Let's talk about marriage. I mean I've been married to my wife for fifteen years, and, you know, I love her, but....

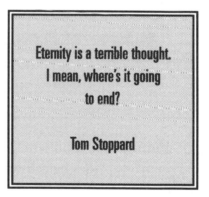

Eternity is a terrible thought.
I mean, where's it going
to end?

Tom Stoppard

The hard fact of the matter is that even with our brief life spans, a high percentage of married couples don't make it for the duration anyway. On the other hand, some couples do celebrate their fiftieth and more anniversaries. There is a danger that we could run out of precious materials and objects to signify future milestones. Your 500th iridium anniversary? The tri-centennial quark anniversary?

Marriage is an area where an immortal society will perhaps work out some new rules of the game. Contract marriages for a fixed number of years, renewable with consent of both parties, would, for instance, be one option. You might wind up remarrying the same person a number of times with other partners scattered in between. And, like boredom, divorce will probably always be with us. It should be no worse a problem in an immortal society than currently, unless you worry about how many times you've been divorced. A three hundred time loser?

> **One reason people get divorced is that they run out of gift ideas.**
>
> **Robert Byrne**

Family could present another interesting dilemma. My mother prides herself on the fact that she has memorized the birthdays of each of her four children, sixteen grandchildren and five great-grandchildren. Obviously, remembering even names could get to be a chore if the number of your offspring gets into the hundreds, which could easily happen. The dispersion to space which will have to take place in order to accommodate an immortal and growing population may alleviate this problem. Out of this world, out of mind.

CHAPTER 11

Right Body, Wrong Century: The Prospect of Culture Shock

> The less things change,
> the more they stay
> the same.
>
> Sicilian Proverb

How can I be sure that I'll like the world of the future? It sounds like it's going to be very different from what I'm used to.

It will be, and there's a very real chance that something like culture shock will be experienced by people from our era who find themselves in the age of nanotechnology. There is evidence in the anthropological literature of the difficulties experienced by people of one culture, usually a more primitive one, being thrust into a wholly different culture. If you've ever travelled to a foreign country, however, you don't need to read about culture shock as it's occurred to other people. It can be quite disconcerting to find yourself in a country where the language, the customs, and the basic details of day-to-day living are quite different from your own.

There are really two separate kinds of cases to consider here, one with much more potential for culture shock than the other. The first scenario would involve a person of our era who manages to survive into the era of nanotechnology and cellular repair machines by dint of relative youth, good health, superior longevity genes and the kind of bootstrapping made possible by advances in medical care (as discussed in Chapter 6). For that person, the changes will be gradual in the sense that the person will live through them. Of course, as discussed in Chapter 9, these transformations might be quite disruptive. A survivor might go through changes as profound as those experienced by a civil war veteran who had lived long enough to see electricity, the automobile, and radio become realities—or a veteran of the first world war who survived to see the marvels of computers, television, and man landing on the moon. Such a person might long for the world as it was when he was young, when his initial impressions of the world were being formed. But, by dint of having lived through the changes, the person might experience something more like culture longing or nostalgia rather than culture shock.

And perhaps you, surviving to the era of nanotechnology, might long for the smell of engine exhausts on a hot sunny day, the stuffed-head misery of a good old-fashioned cold, or the frenzied crush of an overloaded subway car. No? Ah, perhaps you're ready for the future.

> **Progress might have been**
> **all right once,**
> **but it went on too long.**
>
> **Ogden Nash**

A more severe problem is likely to occur among those who will lose consciousness in our present era and regain it in the age of nanotechnology. (How this will be accomplished is discussed in the next section of the book. For now, just be a good sport and assume it happens. OK?) These people will go from our current Earth-bound era of disease, aging, poverty and pollution—to one in which they awaken young, healthy, and immortal. They will find themselves in a society which has vast abundances and cheap space travel...a whole new world.

It is not possible to predict details at such a remove in time, but it may well be that those who take on the responsibility of awakening the sleepers will also help them ease into the new society. This could well be a lengthy process, but when one is immortal that matters little. The main goal to be accomplished during such a period will be to help those who were suspended to develop culturally appropriate expectations. It is incorrect expectations which lead to many of the problems of adapting to a new society (Storti, 1990).

One way to ease the problem of culture shock, a way which could be readily accomplished in the era of nanotechnology, would be to create enclaves. These enclaves could be either deliberately set aside or spontaneously generated. They would be places where people who are not comfortable with the modern society, who long for a different lifestyle from that provided by the fruits of nanotechnology, could reside in quite different surroundings. With more of the earth's surface available for habitation, with inexpensive space travel, and in particular with space habitats economically built through nanotechnology, such enclaves could be large, self-sustaining, and quite interesting places to live or visit.

The whole reawakening and cultural adaptation process for those being brought forward into the era of nanotechnology might reasonably take place in an enclave. Those reawakened might work their way through a variety of environments. These environments would start out closely approximating the person's original culture and then gradually introduce more and more elements of the current culture until the adaptation process was completed. Depending on the number of people to be awakened and the amount of cultural change to be overcome, such an enclave might be a large and long lasting enterprise.

Examples of cultural enclaves exist in our own current society, witness the Amish who cling to the technology and lifestyle of an earlier time. Religious orders such as that of the Trappist monks provide another example of a society within a society which operates in quite different ways and meets some unconventional needs. Given the peculiarities of the human mind, one likely candidate for an enclave in the era of nanotechnology would be one where humans would exist without the benefit of cellular repair nanomachines in their bodies. This would comprise a "natural man" enclave where one could be born, and for sure die, just as some deity or spokesperson ordained.

Any enclave, no matter how faithful a copy of your era, may well lack one important ingredient—family and friends. Waking up in some distant future and finding no loved ones, no friends there with you, is a daunting thought. Trying to convince others to join you in the future is an obvious step one can take to try to forestall this problem. Even if your efforts are successful, though, there is no guarantee that some problem or another might not prevent those you are most fond of from joining you. So, what then?

When you came into this world you necessarily came with family members attached, at least a mother and a father. Some of those reading this book, though, may have never known their birth parents and have been brought up as orphans or adoptees. For others, who once had parents, that status will have changed, parents will have passed on. Therefore, waking up in the future with no biological parents present won't represent a change of status for some.

If you are currently a junior member of a large, close family, the chances that many of those senior family members will join you in the future are quite slender. So those family relationships may not be possible for you in the future. And what about your descendants? Again, they may or may not become convinced to join you. In the future if you want to build another family, to have children, you will be able to do that. They won't be the children you have now, but at least that type of relationship will be possible for you if you so desire.

What of friends? The same arguments apply. They may or may not join you. If you have the capability of making and keeping friends in your current life, there is no reason to suppose you will lose this ability when you awaken in the future. You should be able to develop a new set of friends to replace those who are no longer on the scene. It may have taken you a lifetime to develop and build the friendship bonds you now feel, but you'll have many lifetimes to build similar bonds in the future. A natural pool to draw upon for these new friendships of the future will be among those who have made the transition from the current world to the world of the future. You are bound to have many things in common, including the foresight which made it possible for you to satisfy your desire to see the future.

All of this is not meant to minimize the problem of future shock or the importance of family and friends. They are indeed serious issues to consider. The question, though, is whether a consideration of those issues would lead one to reject the prospect of immortality.

No discussion of strategies for adjusting to a culture would be complete without mention of the most extreme strategy, suicide. With some fluctuation, the suicide rate for humans across cultures seems to hover around one percent. If this propensity to end life is built into the human organism, it is likely to be a factor in the future also. Immortality will be a choice, not a sentence, and some may choose otherwise.

CHAPTER 12

"True" Immortality Versus Death As A Rare Event

> Immortality is the only cause you can't die for.
>
> **Heathcote Williams**

Are you sure you should be using the word immortality? *I can see how nanotechnology and cell repair machines could lead to very healthy people and perhaps no disease, but that doesn't mean you're going to live forever—there are always accidents.*

Immortality is sometimes used to mean "enduring." Authors and other artists are described as "immortal," as are their works of art, if they have been around for several hundred years. I could quibble and say that if Shakespeare's work has been around long enough to be deemed "immortal," then nanotechnology will be able to preserve you long enough for you to be immortal. But, let's not quibble. I mean more than that. Drexler himself, however, agrees with you and says that the use of the term *immortality* to describe the effects of nanotechnological cell repair is incorrect (Drexler, 1986, p.138). In Chapter 16 of this book you will find a discussion of a technique which uses nanotechnology to repair damage to the brain of someone who has been frozen. In order to deal with the question of whether immortality is the right term to use, we'll have to delve into that repair technology a bit.

First, let me repeat that if by immortality you truly mean forever then there is no problem as long as the universe is in a steady state and unending. If, however, the universe might one day come to an end in the opposite of the big bang (the big suck?), which is one of the leading contenders for the history of the universe, then no one and no thing can be immortal. On the other hand, one can argue that without a universe time has no meaning. So, *immortal* might be taken to mean "lasting until the end of the universe." If so, I believe a logical argument could be made that what is being discussed here is true immortality.

In order to support that bold assertion, I'm going to have to discuss how memory is stored in the brain, a somewhat technical subject but very relevant to the discussion at hand. The brain weighs three to four pounds and contains about 100 billion neurons or brain cells. These cells are interconnected in a vast web and are the physical embodiment of our ability to see, hear, taste, think, dream, remember...to be conscious, reasoning animals. Research has shown that memory "appears to involve a sequence of molecular changes at specific locations in systems of neurons" (Alkon, 1989, p.42). Alkon further states that memory "...is represented and stored by a physical pattern of branching and of synaptic contacts..." (1989, p.46).

If the structure of the brain, the neurons and their interconnections, is disturbed, the memory that structure encodes is disturbed. If the structure stays intact, the memory stays intact. As people age they commonly develop an inability to recall something they are positive that they know, the "tip of the tongue" phenomenon. Later, they are very likely to be able to remember the item. The problem consists not of a loss of memory, a change of structure, but rather the ability to accurately and quickly access those structures.

The mechanisms underlying this difficulty are still subject to investigation, but it seems that as long as the structure is there the memory is there. Alzheimers disease, the ultimate forgetting problem, plays its havoc by physically changing the structure of the brain cells and their connections (Selkoe, 1992). In fact, a post mortem examination of the brain is how the ultimate diagnosis of Alzheimers is made.

OK, OK, so what does this have to do with immortality?

Well, if you remember, the contention of this book is that you essentially *are* your memories and personality. If your memories have a structural basis in the brain, then by extrapolation so do other factors of your personality. My argument is that if those memories (in this general sense) can be made immortal, then you can be made immortal.

So how does nanotechnology make my memories immortal? How is it going to help if I'm killed in an accident?

For our purposes there are basically two different kinds of fatal accidents, those in which only your body is damaged and those in which your brain (or both your brain and body) is damaged. Let's examine the first type of accident.

Body Destroyed, Brain Intact

If significant portions of your body are destroyed in some fashion, but your brain is intact, nanotechnology can be used to keep you alive. Your survival will be ensured by growing a new body for you, a clone. The DNA in each cell of your body contains a blueprint of how your body is constructed. Nanotechnology can be used to follow that blueprint and build a new body just like the one that was damaged. It will be a duplicate of your old body, but without any traces of anything that happened to you since you were born. These post-birth traces include such things as injuries, surgery and scars, but also include any information, any memorics, you gained after birth.

> Every man's memory is his
> private literature.
>
> Aldous Huxley

Unless we can restore your memories, you will be an adult-sized infant. So, once the new body is grown (without a brain), your preserved, undamaged brain containing all your memories ("you") will be inserted into the new body and—hey, presto—you're still alive and kicking.

In order for nanotechnology to help you survive, though, the structures of your brain must remain unchanged. We are supposing that your accident leaves your brain untouched, but damages your body sufficiently to cause death. In that case, the blood supply to your brain will be shut off, and after some time the brain will begin to decay. To ensure your survival, then, that decay of your brain must be halted before you begin to lose your memories. The brain must be preserved in some sort of biostasis while your new body is grown.

For now, we'll leave the question of exactly how the decay of your brain might be halted to be answered later. You'll see that there are several possible methods.

Brain Destroyed

A more difficult situation arises if the fatal accident destroys your brain. How can you survive if your memories are destroyed? To see how, think of the nanomachines which will be placed in your body and which will access every cell of your body, including your brain cells, as mapping explorers. What they can map and document can be created anew if need be.

You can think of your brain as a three-dimensional pattern in which all of your memories are stored. Such a pattern can be mapped. Granted it would be a very complex map with billions of bits of information, but in principle it can be done. This is just the sort of thing which computers, nano or otherwise, excel at.

Given the capability for self-replicating nanoassemblers, the production of billions of mapping and exploring nanomachines and nanocomputers is not a difficult task at all. So, imagine that the nanomachines report the exact three dimensional location of each molecule, each nerve ending, in your brain and that this information, all the billion bits of it, is safely stored somewhere outside your body.

In the same place, we'll also store your DNA code either as information or simply as a scrap of material from your body—a strand of hair will do. Now, we go back to the scenario where your brain was destroyed and perhaps your body along with it. Our concern here is for the brain because that is where your memories, "you," reside. By mapping the structure of your brain, we've done what in computer terminology is called a "backup." At the point where the mapping was made you "backed up" all your memories. If your brain is destroyed sometime after that in an accident—crushed, burned, lost at sea or in space—then you and your intact memories can be restored up to the point of your last backup. The DNA will be used to grow a new body, the structure of the brain will be set to the pattern that was stored, and you are in business again.

But how do I know it will really be "me"? Memory is one thing but how about being consciously aware and not just some pattern that was in storage while my new body was grown?

Mind used to be regarded as something immaterial and separate from the brain, but "most neuroscientists now believe that all aspects of mind, including...consciousness or awareness are likely to be explainable...as the behavior of large sets of interacting neurons" (Crick and Koch, 1992). Thus, if we preserve the pattern of those neurons and their interconnections, "you" will be restored. All you will have lost will be whatever memories accrued between the time of your last backup and the time of your death. And, as with people who operate computer machinery, some of whom are better at doing backups than others, how much data you lose will depend on how frequently you do the backups.

OK, but I could still say that that's not true immortality, even as far-out and science-fiction sounding as it is— and yes, I remember, good science fiction is based on plausible assumptions. The reason it's still not true immortality is that the place where you've got your brain pattern and your DNA code stored, that could be destroyed, too. Then where are you? Dead!

Yes, that's true. So now let's get a little more elaborate, take advantage of one of the other features that the coming of nanotechnology will offer, namely practical space travel. If you are truly paranoid about your continued existence, then it would be prudent to store multiple backups in different locations, just as computer operators do who are serious about preserving their data. A fire can destroy a building and destroy both a computer and its backed up data. So, on some regular basis, prudent computer operators take their backup data to some other location and store them. You could do the same thing with the backup of your brain.

In fact, you could store your backup in multiple locations on earth and put a copy in near-earth orbit if you're really worried about bizarre large scale accidents. You could also put a copy on some other planet or astcroid in the solar system. To carry this idea to its ultimate expression, if the thought of the sun going nova is keeping you awake at nights, you could send a backup copy to some other star system on a regular basis. If word reached the remote star system that all your other backup copies had been destroyed, you could be reconstituted. Clearly, given the amount of time necessary for travel to another star system, you would be missing considerably more of your recent memories under this scenario. Still, the memories you have as of the last backup sent to the stars will be yours. That version of you will still be alive. Ergo, true immortality.

> **Death, not space,**
> **is the final frontier.**
>
> **Greg Palmer**

Some people are now talking of "upload" capabilities as providing a form of immortality. The notion is to take your brain pattern (stored as electronic information) and load, or "upload," it into a computer. You would then continue your conscious existence as a self-aware computer. If that computer was then implanted in a clone of your body and you couldn't distinguish the difference between your new existence and your old one, this upload form of immortality would not differ from the one outlined above. If, however, you don't have a body or if your self awareness is qualitatively different, then I would argue that you have not achieved immortality, but an imitation of it. Call me a narrow-minded old fogy if you want.

CHAPTER 13

Powerful Technologies, Powerful Dangers: Avoiding A World of Slime

> The world is populated in the main by people who should not exist.
>
> Bernard Shaw

Just because it's possible to do something, doesn't mean that you should do it. Do you really think it's a good idea to keep everyone alive forever? How about the bad guys, what if this stuff was available when Hitler was

*around? What about Kadafy, what about Sadaam
Hussein? There are some really terrible people out there,
and I'm sure more will be born in the future.*

The question raises a rather profound issue which
involves not just the few truly evil people whom we can
think of whose lives we wouldn't want extended, but a
very general principle. If we take Shaw at his word there
were a lot of people he thought shouldn't be alive at all, let
alone be granted immortality. Probably there are people in
your life you'd just as soon not have around forever, even
if *you* could be around that long.

To see the nature of the issue, let's assume first of all
that nanotechnology is available. Let's also assume that
cellular repair nanotechnology is as inexpensive as it
seems likely to be. (Remember the three dollar LCD
wristwatch.) Now, let's assume that there is some wicked
person who is a test case for us. This incarnation of evil
is on his death bed, and we think he is a person whose
life should not be extended. My question is this: is there
a moral difference between withholding cellular repair
nanotechnology from that person and, in the present
day, executing such a person?

I believe the answer is no. There is no moral difference between the two actions. Society is doing the same
thing in either case, which is to deny the person any
chance at further life. To say that some people will not
deserve immortality is the moral equivalent of saying
that there are currently people who do not deserve to be

alive. While I grant you the right to hold this opinion, I'm not sure that society would consider it acceptable behavior for you to go out and murder some of those undeserving people. Many of the world's societies, of course, do have procedures for executing people who have transgressed and the same kind of rules could and probably should be applied to the granting or continuance of immortality.

I believe that in the future it will not be acceptable to withhold cellular repair nanotechnology from anyone arbitrarily . So where does that leave us with true villains such as Hitler, serial killers, and the like? It would seem to leave us just where we've always been. They are the responsibility of saner, better people than themselves to contain, to deal with. The fact that, if unexecuted, they are likely to be around nearly forever may seem discouraging, but in point of fact you will be around for just as long, so that factor is counterbalanced.

Before we examine some possible solutions, we need to be sure we're covering the true scope of the problem. So far we've been talking about a few very malignant people of a highly visible nature. The same problem occurs on a smaller scale of evil, but over a much broader number of people, when we talk about simply criminal behavior. People who violate the legal precepts of society, who do things outside the bounds and infringe upon the rights of others, robbers, thieves, murderers, etc., must be considered also. In the United States about four tenths of a percent of our population is in prison. That represents just over one million people. As our sentencing laws get stricter, with such measures as "three strikes and you're out", a growing percentage of those prisoners will be there for life. Are we faced with the prospect of sending people to prison for life when their lives are unending? What a burden on society that would be. And how much more dramatic executing a criminal would be when the execution is depriving the criminal of not forty or fifty years of life, but of untold centuries.

There are no simple solutions to this problem. It is a complex ethical-moral question and provides an illustration of one of the consequences of nanotechnology which needs exposure and debate in the public arena before the capability is fully upon us. It will be much tougher to deal with this issue when it actually becomes possible to give someone cellular repair devices to allow him to live forever, and murderer's row is full up. Humans being humans, that is probably exactly when the debate will take place, but one can hope.

Though there are no simple answers, there may be some mitigating factors which will help us deal with the problem of common criminals. Criminal and deviant behavior will probably always be with us as long as we're humans. To the extent that such behavior is driven by economic factors, though, one could hypothesize that in an age of abundance there would be less reason, less emotionally driven reason, less rage, to provide the motive force for the criminal behavior.

On the other hand such behavior may not be driven by the absolute level of your possessions, but by the gap between what you have and what your rich neighbors have. The United States, for instance, is one of the richest countries on the planet, and also has one of the highest crime rates, particularly for violent crimes. Since in all of man's ages differences in wealth accumulation have existed, the age of nanotechnology is not likely to be any different. If so, "gap-driven" crime will still be with us.

It may also be that at some point in the future, people will be granted the right to dose their bodies with whatever mind-altering substances they want. In other words, drugs or their nanotechnology equivalents may become legalized. If so, the economic incentive for the smuggling, distribution, and sale of illegal drugs will no longer exist. A high percentage of crime in the United States can be tied directly to trafficking in drugs, which can be a very lucrative though dangerous profession. If drug trafficking is no longer lucrative because it is no longer illegal, if drugs are readily available, there will be no economic motive for the bulk of the people now engaged in such activity to continue. Granted, there may be some other problems society has to deal with, but the tradeoff would be well worth it.

Let us assume, though, that there is some irreducible minimum of deviant behavior that economic factors do not affect. Let us further assume that the only way to deal with the behavior is to modify the people engaging in the behavior, or to remove them from society. It is possible, and very likely, that as we map the structure of the human brain more and more types of deviant behavior will be found to be physically caused. For instance, it is already known that the mental illnesses of schizophrenia and mania are marked by biochemical and structural changes in the brain (Gershon and Rieder, 1992). Drugs to treat these diseases work on the brain cells at the molecular level. Since these kinds of problems can be physically corrected, the same may be true for various categories of anti-social behavior.

An example of such a physical cause for criminal behavior was recently reported (Richardson, 1993). A genetic defect on the X chromosome has been identified as the cause of violently aggressive behavior by several generations of men in one family. Such research leads to the hope that someday soon we will be able to address and cure the basic causes of many such problems, rather than incarcerating or otherwise removing people from society.

As with other aspects of the technology, however, capability brings moral dilemma. If you can determine physically what causes a certain kind of behavior and if society deems that behavior inappropriate, do we really have the right to go in and physically modify the brain structure of the offending person? It seems quite clear when we're talking about child molestation or serial killers. It is not so clear, and getting into the danger zone, when we're talking about someone who is just different than the rest of society, a hermit for instance or someone who likes to skip backward through the park singing nonsense syllables and eating dandelions.

It would be safe to assume that there will be some anti-social behaviors not subject to physical correction, and some behaviors which are subject to correction but for which societal intervention is not deemed appropriate. Thus, we'll still be faced with the problem of dealing with some people who are a burden to society in one way or another.

Various possibilities for dealing with this sub-population exist. One such would be to use the current system of imprisonment. It would seem reasonable that the percentage of the population represented by such people would be sufficiently reduced that they would not be a large burden. In addition, with the physical abundance provided by nanotechnology, keeping such people in relative comfort should not be all that expensive a proposition. But how would we determine an equitable sentence, particularly for the incorrigible criminal? A life sentence would be a very cruel prospect for an immortal to face, since it would mean that he or she would be locked up in prison forever.

A perhaps more humane possibility would be to designate some area off the planet as an enclave, probably a guarded enclave, for such people—a dumping ground if you will. It would be the future's equivalent of the way Australia was used by England back in the early days. This future enclave could be on the surface of another planet in our solar system, in an artificial space habitat, or perhaps in another star system. Such treatment might also be judged somewhat cruel. Locking a bunch of societal misfits up together and letting them sort things out could lead to a brutal anarchy. Taking away their lives or incarcerating them forever seems little better, however. This is not an area where an elegant, easy solution appears likely.

So, to sum up, 1) criminals may always be with us, 2) yes, we could withhold immortality, but 3) it is the moral equivalent of killing them. We in the United States don't kill very many prisoners today, and the rest of the industrialized nations kill even fewer. I doubt that in the future we will do things very differently.

Besides problems about what to do with criminals, what other predicaments is nanotechnology likely to get us into?

Technological progress is like an axe in the hands of a pathological criminal.

Albert Einstein

Any technology capable of ushering in an era of material abundance, space travel, freedom from disease and aging, and immortality for the human race, is clearly very powerful. However, as with nuclear energy, there is a dark side, a dangerous side to nanotechnology. These dangers can be categorized as either inadvertent or deliberate. Perhaps the most frightening inadvertent misuse of nanotechnology thus far imagined is a scenario of runaway, self-replicating assemblers which quickly turn the earth into a world of slime, or goo, or whatever nasty substance fires your imagination. The fear is somewhat akin to that which preceded the first atomic explosion when some thought it might trigger a chain reaction which would destroy the earth.

Though Drexler was the first one to discuss the nanoassembler "run amuck" danger, he has since reconsidered (Drexler, 1986, "Afterword"). Keeping in mind that self-replicating assemblers will be carefully programmed by humans, there is no real reason to believe that these assemblers would "run wild." Their programming could be set up so that they stay within certain defined boundaries. Even though they might have the capability of essentially free-ranging and finding their own energy source, they will not be programmed that way.

Computers in our current world do not reprogram themselves and commit malignant acts, and there is no reason to think that nanomachines would either. The analogy Drexler uses is that nanomachines would be no more likely to run wild in that way than an automobile is likely to go out and start searching for its own gasoline.

Other accidental misuses of nanotechnology depend more on human error than on malignant machines.

Take, for instance, a nanoseed, which is simply some assemblers combined with nanocomputers programmed to eventually create whatever device you want. Imagine that this seed is designated for disassembling mine tailings in an environmental clean-up effort. Imagine that the seed is inadvertently placed in a different environment, an environment where some of the same materials it is supposed to disassemble are located in a finished product form, such as a warehouse containing appliances. It is conceivable that the nanomachines could disassemble the appliances into their component molecules, rather than the mine tailings it was designed to handle. Such a scenario seems unlikely, but humans have been known to commit some very unlikely mistakes with or without the aid of high technology. The bottom line is that nanotechnology like any technology must be handled with adequate safeguards to prevent disruptive, and perhaps even life-threatening, accidents from happening.

> **An idea that is not dangerous is unworthy of being called an idea at all.**
>
> **Oscar Wilde**

The dangers likely to occur from inadvertent misuses of nanotechnology, however, pale by comparison with the more serious threat of deliberate misuse. It is instructive to note that the phrase is "beating their swords into plowshares" rather than the reverse. The implication is that the sword was there first. It seems that often man's first use of a new technology is to create weapons with it. This may also be true of nanotechnology, and the weapons which can be created with nanotechnology promise to be legion, lethal and frightening.

Consider first conventional weapons. Now think of nanoassemblers replicating themselves and rapidly building a vast arsenal of these weapons, perhaps with improved materials and designs. A group or country with nanotechnology capability could become a military power, at least in terms of weapons, in a very short period of time.

Nanoseeds, dropped from the air or smuggled into an area, whose purpose is to destroy crops, water supplies, human flesh, or other weapons, are also conceivable. Keeping in mind the molecular size of nano devices it would be virtually impossible to detect them through any macro means. Thus it would be very easy to smuggle them wherever you wanted either inside humans or within inanimate objects being transported around the world.

At a more personal level, someone with the knowledge and capability could make an extremely effective poison using nanotechnology. A poison could be made which would do its work and then disassemble itself into harmless substances. These substances could then be flushed out of the system or even dissipated through into the air, leaving behind no trace of their presence.

As mentioned earlier, nanotechnology could also be used to make drug-like substances which would make designer drugs seem like clumsy, crude approximations of the real thing. It would be virtually impossible to stop the smuggling of such drugs in nanoseed form.

No misuse of nanotechnology, of course, will be very simple and straightforward. We are talking about very sophisticated technology. But the past has shown that there are always people with good technological capability who can be tempted to create whatever horrors the mind of man can conceive. They will do it either from motives of personal profit or in the service of some "cause."

In essence, then, nanotechnology, like any technology, can be used for purposes good or ill. Is that a reason to try to stop its development? There are two answers to that question. One is that the benefits far outweigh the potential dangers, although those dangers can be frightening to contemplate. The other, more potent, answer is that it will be virtually impossible to stop the development of nanotechnology. As argued earlier, the beginnings of nanotechnology are in place, they are well known, and development is taking place in a variety of fields and in several countries. At this stage it is better to identify and recognize the dangers, do everything in our power to minimize their potential to cause problems, and move forward.

***

Undoubtedly, there are arguments against immortality that the book has not covered, but I think we have touched on the major ones. Before moving on to the next section of the book, let's summarize where we've been so far. The book has argued that physical immortality is possible, that the human body is a machine which, like other machines, can be kept repaired and functioning indefinitely. The likely mechanism for repairing the body at the cellular level will come through nanotechnology. Nanomachines capable of rapid, inexpensive replication will be able to monitor and repair each of the billions of cells in your body.

Some of the more serious societal problems which the real prospect of immortality raises have been discussed. It has been shown that the cheap mass-production capabilities of nanotechnology could alleviate many of these problems including the availability of material goods, living space, food, and the problems of pollution. The future world of nanotechnology, in fact, should be a very interesting and wondrous place to live in.

But...how are you going to get there? Chapter 6 promised that the question of how to get from the "here" of our current world to the "there" of immortality would be answered later. It is time now to move on to that answer.

GETTING
FROM HERE
TO THERE

CHAPTER 14

Narrowing the Gap: Pushing Your Life Span and Nanotechnology

Life is uncertain; eat dessert first.

Bumper Sticker

So, here you are. The thought of living in a perfectly functioning body which does not age, in an era of material abundance appeals to you. You are convinced that cellular repair nanotechnology will inevitably be developed, though no one knows when. So, what do you do about it? Just forget it and hope for the best? Spend all your time in desperate longing, glued to the media, scanning for the most recent scientific advances? Or would you like to do something more rational, more proactive? From a logical point of view, there are three different kinds of actions you can take to help you reach the time when immortality will be feasible. One possibility is to do whatever you can to help push the advance of nanotechnology. Another, is to do your best to increase your own natural longevity by keeping in good health. Finally, assuming you don't win that battle, you can make arrangements to be put in biostasis until such time as the battle has been won.

Pushing the Process

One person is unlikely to have much of an impact on advancing the time when nanotechnology comes to fruition. But, like many tiny rivulets which eventually become a mighty river, even small, seemingly inconsequential actions by individuals can join together to make a true difference. Of course, if you are a scientist or engineer working in nanotechnology-related areas, and can turn your attention to things which will further the goal of reaching nanotechnology, you would be taking the most direct kind of action one could hope to take. A student might think about entering a discipline which is related to nanotechnology, if not nanotechnology itself.

There are now courses in nanotechnology, but, as of this writing, no institutions which offer a nanotechnology major.

Even the rest of us, who have no scientific or technological background, who are locked into other careers, can have some impact. One of the easiest and perhaps most beneficial things we can do is to join the Foresight Institute. As mentioned earlier this institute is devoted to spreading the word about nanotechnology and helping society anticipate the many changes which will take place and the many decisions which will need to be made. You will find information on the Foresight Institute in the Resources section at the back of the book.

Another way in which individuals can have some impact is through the political process by which the funding for scientific projects is carried out. Keeping in tune with such things, and staying in touch with your elected representatives in the government to express your interest in having nanotechnology and related technologies fostered may have an impact. Again, the impact by any particular individual may not be large; but if enough of us are hammering away, we may significantly advance the coming of nanotechnology by simply helping channel scientific research into the right paths.

Finally, just talking to people about nanotechnology can have a positive effect. The more people who know about the possibilities, the more momentum we can gain. You might even go hog wild and write a book!

Pushing the Body

As I discussed earlier, getting yourself from here to there will be more likely if you are young and in good health. All of the things you've heard about and read about *ad nauseam* which can help lengthen your life span are relevant here. The statistics, though, can get a little discouraging. Recent conclusions from a long-term study suggest that regular exercise can add a whopping eight months to your life span. Now, according to the researchers that's a large jump, but from an individual's point of view eight months doesn't seem like a very big deal. Of course, the exercise will probably also increase what some people call your health span, the amount of time in which you are active and in good health, by a much longer period of time. Another way to think about the issue is to speculate that during that extra eight months you've granted yourself, somebody may just make the discovery that will keep you alive for another eight months, allowing you to bootstrap your way through to the future.

When all is said and done, however, all of these kinds of efforts may not be enough—push may come to shove.

By the time a man is ready to die, he is fit to live.

Ed Howe

Chapter 15

When Push Comes To Shove: Biostasis

> Eventually everybody has to die, except Elvis.
>
> Dave Barry

No matter how hard you try or how much we might wish it would be otherwise, chances are it is going to take longer for cellular repair nanotechnology to come about than you or I have. We don't know for sure, of course, but you'd better not bet too much on the optimistic side. Part of the problem is simply that nanotechnology might be less than a decade away, but nanotechnology capable of cellular repair, mature nanotechnology, is surely further away than that and maybe significantly further away.

We need to look at some cold, hard facts here having to do with the human body. Those facts are that the body contains hundreds of kinds of cells, hundreds of thousands of different kinds of molecules, and hundreds of billions of cells. The repairs these cells need might be quite complex. Mind you, I'm not backing off here and saying that cellular repair nanomachines are not possible. I'm simply saying that it will probably be the most complex application of nanotechnology, and therefore likely to be developed considerably later than other applications.

As a prudent person, then, who is interested in becoming immortal, you would want to look beyond what we've already discussed. You would look for a way to hang around until cellular repair nanotechnology is available. Essentially, what you'd like to accomplish is to go into a kind of time warp and come out on the other side when the technology is available. In practical terms, you want to enter what can be called *biostasis,* a state in which biological processes are suspended. You don't want to enter that state until you've lived out your current life, but entering a time warp at that point would be most convenient.

In principle, biostasis would refer to any technique for attaining the desired goal of stopping the biological decay process. In practice, there is only one method being used at this time to achieve biostasis for humans. That process is freezing. We need to make some important distinctions here because they will be necessary to help you sort out different people's opinions about the topics we will be discussing.

The distinctions have to do with the science of freezing things. In general, the technique we are interested in is known as *cryogenics*. Cryogenics is concerned with studying the properties of matter at very low temperatures. When the matter being studied at low temperatures is living tissue, the area is referred to as *cryobiology*. Practical applications of cryobiology include the storage of frozen, viable tissues and organs for later transplantation. Freezing sperm and using them later to fertilize an ovum is one example of such an application.

Finally, when the organism being frozen is a complete human being, the term that is applied is *cryonics*. Strangely, from my point of view, while cryogenics and cryobiology are respected and respectable disciplines, cryonics is not. There are several reasons for this as we will see. You should know up-front, though (if you don't already have an opinion gathered from the media or other sources), that cryonics is a tainted term to many.

CHAPTER 16

Cryonics:
A Chilling Tale
of Suspense

> I'm not afraid to die.
> I just don't want
> to be there
> when it happens.
>
> Woody Allen

Cryonics consists of freezing a human body which is then stored at a very cold temperature to await later resuscitation. Cryonics is both simple to understand and very controversial. Much of the controversy relates to the fact that cryonics represents a two-part problem, the second part of which is beyond the power of current technology to solve.

The first part of the problem is how to freeze a human body. The basic procedure is relatively straightforward. You simply place the body in liquid nitrogen, which has a temperature of -196^0 centigrade. The body will be solidly frozen and will stay that way, without decay, for as long as the liquid nitrogen is maintained. The actual process used is quite a bit more elaborate than just stated, but the essentials are the same. Research is still being conducted on various ways to improve the technique, and will be discussed later. For now, few would argue that we don't know how to freeze a human body.

The second part of the cryonics problem is the source of all the controversy, namely how to thaw out and revive the frozen person. That part of the problem has not been solved yet and probably won't be for some time. The cryobiologists who are attempting to freeze and then reanimate living organisms have not been able to do so with complete success. Because of that failure most cryobiologists do not think cryonics is a valid procedure. They feel the damage done to the body by the freezing process cannot be repaired.

They are right as far as current technology goes, but short-sighted, I and others believe, regarding the potential of nanotechnology to make the necessary repairs. Their prejudice is so strong that cryobiologists risk expulsion from professional organizations for working in, or publishing in, the field of cryonics. As I said, the reputation of cryonics is tainted.

Because the ability of nanotechnology to repair and reanimate a frozen body is central to the thesis of this book, to your becoming immortal, it is worth exploring in some detail. Though most cryobiologists have accepted the professional muzzle put on them, not all have. I highly recommend that you read a fascinating, albeit somewhat technical, account by a cryobiologist of how nanotechnology might be used in a step-by-step fashion to repair freezing and other damage to a suspended body and then to reanimate that body. The article, by Dr. Gregory Fahy, is "A 'Realistic' Scenario for Nanotechnological Repair of the Frozen Human Brain" and appears in *Cryonics* (1993). I'll discuss the article in a little more detail later.

History

Cryonics has what some would call a checkered past. Since it represents the current best way of achieving biostasis and helping you to become immortal, I think it would be wise to briefly describe that past. We'll look at the history of the movement, including some of the events which achieved public notoriety and detracted from its reputation.

We live in an era of unsurpassed technological wonders. It was perhaps inevitable that someone would have the vision to suggest that those wonders might be applied to the human life span. The notion suggested, as we have seen, was that it might be possible to preserve a person who had just died in such a way that he could later be revived in an era of greater technological expertise. The person who had that vision, who wrote the book which captured the imagination of many, is Robert C.W. Ettinger. At the time he was a physics professor at a small Michigan college, and the book was *The Prospect of Immortality* published in 1964. This book was actually preceded by another by N. During called *Immortality, Scientifically, Now* (During, 1962). But since During's book was never issued in quantity, Ettinger is seen as the founder of the cryonics movement.

Following publication of Ettinger's book, several groups were formed to carry out in fact what Ettinger was suggesting in principle. The first cryonics society was founded in New York in 1965, and the first human was frozen in January of 1967 (Smith, 1983). (His name is Dr. James Bedford, and he is still suspended awaiting reanimation (Perry, 1994)). The groups met with some initial success and were able to attract both like-minded people and public notice. Some of the members of the early cryonics societies appeared on talk shows and had active publicity campaigns to generate interest in their organizations. Things appeared to be going great guns for a while. For an interesting account of one of these groups and interviews with the people who made up the group you can read *Cryonics: A Sociology Of Death And Bereavement* (Sheskin, 1979).

Two sorts of problems beset these groups after their initial success. One set of problems was of a practical nature, and the other had to do with basic human motivations. The practical problems revolved around money. There was no single accepted plan or mechanism for paying for the cryonic suspension and upkeep costs, so a number of different avenues, willy-nilly, were explored by the groups. This led to some of the negative publicity the groups received. One payment method that was tried early on was simply pay as you go. The problem was that once a person was cryonically suspended he or she was no longer doing the paying, their surviving family members were. Given that there is an indefinite period of time in which payments have to be made, this turned into a rather shaky financial arrangement. One of the people running a cryonics organization was accused of being heartless because if a family began falling behind on the maintenance payments, he would ask if they wanted him to let the suspended person thaw out and rot. Not a pretty picture.

There were also storage problems. The same group discussed above began by storing capsules containing the suspended people in a cemetery building. When that arrangement was terminated by the cemetery, a mad scramble ensued to find an appropriate storage facility. There is also an incident recorded where a lawsuit was successfully brought against the operators of a cryonics facility which, in the mid 1970's, allowed nine bodies to thaw out. Obviously the cryonics gamble did not pay off for those nine people.

> The best laid plans of mice
> and men...are about equal.
>
> Unknown

As you will see when we get into the details of making arrangements for cryonic suspension for yourself (if you so desire), things have evolved to a much better state. There is still plenty of room for improvement in all areas, however.

The standard arrangement at the largest cryonics organization currently in existence, The Alcor Life Extension Foundation (see Resources for more information), includes making arrangements for a lump sum bequest to the non-profit organization. Upon your legal death this lump sum pays for the cost of the suspension and the maintenance costs indefinitely into the future, and also pays for the treatment and transportation needed to get you to the cryonics facility when you "deanimate," as they so delicately put it. In addition, while you are still alive there is an annual fee to cover ongoing organizational costs. The lump sum is typically funded through a whole life insurance policy, but obviously could also be a trust fund you set up, assuming you have the wherewithal. All of this will be covered in more detail in a later chapter.

The other area which caused difficulties for the early cryonicists had to do with psychological barriers. One such barrier had to do with intermediate goals. Once a cryonics society was formed and members were meeting, there were few other goals which could be reached in the short term. Essentially the ultimate goal of the society is to play a waiting game. One by one members would go into suspension hoping to meet again at later date. But when that later date would be and—even more importantly I believe—how the reanimation would take place were unknowns. Thus, the early enthusiasm waned. Additionally, I would imagine such normal sorts of club activities as social dances might not have seemed appropriate. What music could one play after all? Pavane For a Dead Princess? Dance Macabre?

Another psychological barrier occurred on a more personal basis. As documented in Sheskin's (1979) book, the members of at least one of the early cryonics societies were initially very stimulated, excited and eager about what they were doing. As a consequence, they told everyone in their social and family circles what they were up to. They were surprised when their ideas met with much resistance and skepticism. They soon discovered that if they spoke of such things very often they would be branded eccentrics at best. It is difficult to remain excited about something when you can't share the excitement with the world at large.

Still another barrier was the lack of certainty as to when the ultimate goal would be reached. If you belong to Big Brothers or Big Sisters, you get associated with a child, you meet with the child. Those are goal completion steps. If you belong to Junior League there are meetings, and there are projects to be completed each year. Goals are met, and the group can take satisfaction in their accomplishments.

With cryonics, the goal is to survive somehow until such time as you can be revived and cured by the medical science of the future. Probably you can contemplate that goal and talk about it only so long before it loses some of its intrinsic interest. Life goes on, other things come up, cryonics groups lose their momentum.

Another factor, mentioned by George P. Smith III (1983), is that the cryonics movement has never had a charismatic leader. Perhaps such a leader would have provided some necessary invigoration. There is evidence that many of these negative factors have changed in recent years, that the cryonics movement has been newly energized. I suspect that the main factor causing this re-invigoration is the advent of nanotechnology. Having a clearly laid out mechanism whereby those frozen can be repaired and reanimated is crucial. Other nanotechnology-driven factors which undoubtedly have a positive impact would include the belief that repair and reanimation will be inexpensive, that many overpopulation problems can be solved, and that those suspended will awaken to a life of high quality.

Figure 2 shows that after years of very slow growth, Alcor experienced a sharp upturn in membership soon after the publication of the first book on nanotechnology in 1986. Where there's hope there's life. An article and an essay contest which ran in Omni magazine (Platt, 1993) also led to a noticeable increase in inquiries and new members for Alcor. The article discussed nanotechnology and cryonics and offered a free suspension for the winner of the essay contest.

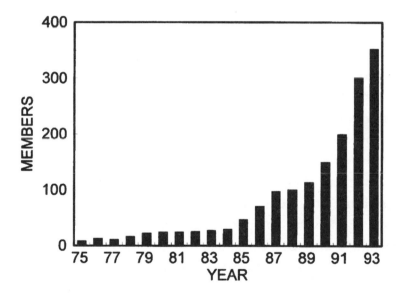

Figure 2. Number of people making arrangements to be suspended by the Alcor Life Extension Foundation for the years 1975–1993. (Data provided courtesy of the Alcor Foundation.)

Where do I find one of these cryonics organizations?

There are six cryonics organizations currently active, one in Arizona, four in California and one in Michigan. You will find complete addresses and phone numbers for each of them, as well as other information, in the Resources section at the back of the book. The six are the Alcor Life Extension Foundation in Scottsdale, Arizona; the American Cryonics Society in Cupertino, California; CryoCare in Culver City, California; the Cryonics Institute in Detroit, Michigan; the International Cryonics Foundation in Stockton, California: and Trans Time Inc. in Oakland, California.

One basic difference between cryonics organizations has to do with whether they are for-profit or non-profit. Alcor, the American Cryonics Society, CryoCare, the Cryonics Institute, and the International Cryonics Foundation are a non-profit organizations. Trans Time, Inc., on the other hand, is a for-profit corporation in which there are a number of stock holders. Alcor performs several functions including information dispersal, research, recovery services (preparing and bringing to the facility members who die), the actual suspension process, and the storage and maintenance of those suspended. The Cryonics Institute and Trans Time also fulfill those functions with the exception that they provide no recovery service; patients must be brought to the facility for suspension.

The American Cryonics Society, CryoCare, and the International Cryonics Foundation perform neither the suspension nor the storage process. They have arrangements with other organizations to carry out suspensions and provide long term storage. All of these kinds of arrangements appear workable. Whether one is better than the other will be a matter of individual judgment and you should contact the different organizations for details on how they operate to find one which best suits your needs..

So what exactly happens during a cryonic suspension?

There are a number of steps in the process, so let's work through an ideal case history. In a later chapter we'll talk about how reality might diverge from that ideal, that is, what kinds of complications and problems might arise. For the purposes of our case study we'll walk through the process with an exemplary character named Lazarus Phoenix, Laz for short. The first step, obviously, is that Laz must belong to a cryonics organization and must have made arrangements to be suspended. Let us suppose that is true and further suppose that Laz joined the Alcor Life Extension Foundation in Scottsdale, Arizona.

Laz lives in the Phoenix area and discovers one not-so-fine day that after living a rich and full life he is suffering from cancer, which has spread throughout his body. Even the most advanced radiation and chemotherapy techniques offer no hope. He has but a short time to live. Laz checks into the hospital when the end is near and makes sure that his physician understands what his wishes are. The recovery team for Alcor knows approximately when

he will die and will be standing by at the hospital. Laz
has resigned himself to departing his current life. Today's
medical science can no longer keep him alive.

As soon as Laz is pronounced legally dead, the Alcor
recovery team assumes his care. The hospital has been
keeping Laz on a heart and lung machine, and now the
recovery team switches him over to their portable life
suspension unit. In addition to keeping his circulation
going, they pack Laz in water ice. Once he is completely
hooked up to the life suspension unit, his temperature is
brought down to a few degrees above freezing for his trip
to the Alcor facility. Both the heart and lung machine
and the cooling are designed to minimize any decay of
Laz's brain cells between the point of legal death and the
completion of the suspension process.

Laz's family members, of course, have been fully
informed of his desires, know what to expect, and are
very supportive. (Remember, we're describing the ideal
situation here). His wife proceeds to the Alcor facility to
witness the suspension. Once at the Alcor facility, cryoprotectant fluids (read human anti-freeze) are introduced into Laz's body to minimize freezing damage. He
is then cooled down over a period of several days to an
ultimate temperature of -196^0 Centigrade and then put
into long term storage. Liquid nitrogen will be used to
keep him at that temperature for years, decades, centuries or however long it takes before Lazarus Phoenix
can be revived to walk the earth again.

> Everything comes if a man
> will only wait.
>
> Benjamin Disraeli

Well, won't our buddy, Laz, decay away if he has to wait decades or centuries?

At the temperature of liquid nitrogen, -196^0, virtually all physical processes have come to a halt. Electrons are barely moving in their orbits. A second's worth of decay at room temperature would take millions of years to occur at -196^0, so Laz will have plenty of time to wait for technology to catch up with his dreams. Of course, from Laz's point of view the passage of time is immaterial. The only factor that will have some impact will be how drastically society and the world changes between the time of his suspension and the time of his reawakening. If it takes twenty years the changes should be easy to absorb. If it takes a hundred years the changes will be substantial—imagine being transported from the world of 1894 to 1994. Obviously, the longer Laz is in suspension the more radical the changes to which he will have to adapt.

Let's back up a minute. Why did Laz have to die before he was suspended? Since he was going to die for sure, wouldn't it have been better to just go ahead and suspend him before any decay had a chance to start?

It would have been better. However, because the suspension process itself will result in death, state laws currently require that the person must be declared legally dead before the cryonic suspension process can start.

Well, I have to admit the whole process sounds a little strange to me. I mean I understand in theory what you're saying. Somebody is dead, you freeze them, and then you bring them back when you can fix them, but I have a hard time with that. Seems like dead is dead. If the person has been declared legally dead...then, what's the point?

Desperate diseases require desperate measures.

Guy Fawkes

I admit, it can seem a little strange. Think about this however. You're viewing death as a singular yes-no event. In fact, death is a process.

What do you mean, a process?

Think about the changes in the legal definition of death that have taken place in recent years. It used to be the case, not too many years ago, that the legal definition of death was the cessation of the heart beat. Once a person's heart stopped beating, they were declared dead. Then more advanced medical knowledge and technology came along such that a stopped heart could be started again. If that restart took place without too much of a time lapse, the person suffered no ill effects. So, a person who once would have been declared legally dead was now alive. Medical science changed, and the legal definition of death changed.

Imagine, if you will, that someone from that earlier time period has just been declared legally dead because his heart stopped. Now imagine that with very little time lapse the body was put in biostasis and then brought forward to the present. In the present, the biostasis is broken, doctors immediately get the heart beating because now we know how to do that, and someone who was legally dead is now alive and kicking. That is the essence of the cryonics argument. The fact that you are declared legally dead in our era does not mean that you could not be revived in a future era with more knowledge.

> Cryonics is an ambulance to
> take a patient to a doctor
> 100 years in the future.
>
> Steve Bridge

In most countries of the world, death is now legally defined by loss of brain function (Wikler, 1993). In fact, however, people have recovered from states in which they had no vital signs and gone on to lead normal lives. Generally they have been children who were submersed in icy cold waters for extended periods of time (Biggart and Bohn, 1990). No heartbeat, no brain wave, but when their body temperature is carefully brought back to normal, the heart functions and so does the brain. So, even our current legal definition of death is shown to be inadequate in certain situations.

Death is a process, not an event. During the process the heart stops, electrical activity in the brain stops, and brain cells decay and lose structure. Just where in the process we say that death has occurred changes as medical science changes. Presumably the legal definition of death will change again in the future as medical science becomes able to cope with conditions from which there is now no recovery. People interested in cryonics differentiate between "legal" death and "memory" or "information theoretic" death. Information theoretic death is what happens when your brain structures have decayed enough that the essential "you," your memories and personality, is gone. So, dead isn't necessarily dead—legal death is not the same as memory death. If the person can be brought back to life some time later with memories and personality intact, suspending them now makes perfectly good sense. That is the hope and the expectation of cryonics.

But, don't the brain cells burst when you freeze somebody? Won't that cause memory death?

This is a popular misconception about what happens when cells are frozen. In fact, ice does not form in cells during ordinary conditions of slow freezing. The ice forms <u>between</u> cells, and the cells actually shrink as water is drawn from them (see *Cryonics,* 1993, Appendix A).

So people really think that once you're frozen solid, and you've been that way for years, you can be revived?

Yes. I mentioned previously Dr. Fahy's description of a hypothetical resuscitation using nanotechnology. The process takes place in a number of stages with different nanomachines having different functions working in sequence. The restoration stages would include stabilizing and mapping the cell structures, removing water and cryoprotectants, establishing a repair network, slow warming, repairing cells, restoring metabolic functions, reversing the effects of disease and age, and, ta da!—awakening. As envisioned by Dr. Fahy, the entire process could take up to a year from start to finish. From the point of view of the person frozen, the amount of time taken is a relatively unimportant issue since he or she will be unconscious throughout the entire process. And remember, the person will wake up cured of whatever physical problems ailed them at the time of suspension and with youth and vigor restored.

> One short sleep past, we wake eternally,
> And Death shall be no more:
> Death, thou shalt die.
>
> John Donne

CHAPTER 17

Many Are Cold
But Few Are Frozen

> Those who welcome death have
> only tried it from the ears up.
>
> **Wilson Mizner**

OK, let's get to the bottom line here. What does it cost to be suspended?

There are a number of costs associated with cryonic suspension. In order to be suspended you first must belong to a cryonics organization and make arrangements. Since the Alcor Foundation is the largest cryonics organization, I'll use their figures for illustration. Costs for all the organizations can be found in the Resources section.

153

Alcor has a sign-up fee of $150. In addition to that there is an annual membership fee of $324. The biggest cost of course is for the actual suspension and then storage of the body. Pricing decisions also take into account the fact that funds will someday be needed to cover reanimation costs. The size of the suspension fee depends on which of two options one takes for being suspended. The first option is whole-body suspension where your entire body is perfused with cryoprotectants and frozen in liquid nitrogen. This procedure at Alcor currently costs $120,000.

The other option, which is becoming increasingly popular, although somewhat controversial, is called neurosuspension and involves the suspension of just the brain. That procedure costs $50,000. Although these sums are obviously substantial, they compare favorably to the costs of current major medical procedures, such as organ transplants. As a practical matter, neurosuspensions typically include the head as well as the brain it contains.

Hold on a minute here. Freeze just my head? Are you serious?

Yes. One of the benefits, as you can see, is the substantially lower cost of both the suspension procedure and the storage costs—$120,000 vs. $50,000. Of course, lower cost is not a reasonable goal if you can't be brought back to life in your own body, but in fact you can be. What you have to keep in mind here is that no one will be revived from a suspended state until medical science is advanced to such a degree that damaged cells can be repaired and the problems that led to suspension in the first place can be cured. The argument of this book is that those goals will be accomplished through nanotechnology.

It will also be possible, using nanotechnology, to take DNA material from the body, including the head, and rebuild the body using the code contained in the DNA. We are reading parts of the DNA code now, and in the future we will be able to read all of it and follow the directions to build a complete body. Nanomachines and assemblers will be able to reconstruct your body according to the instructions contained in your DNA. If that sounds implausible to you, consider how your current body was grown—it started as a single cell and grew according to the DNA instructions contained in that cell.

At the same time that your head is being unfrozen and repaired, a new body will be grown for you, just like your old body except in perfect condition. If, for instance, you had your appendix taken out or other kinds of surgery, that surgery will no longer be in evidence on your new body. DNA code does not contain information about what happened to you after you were born. Your old brain will be placed in your new body. The DNA could be used to grow a new brain too, but it would contain no memories, it would be as blank as a new-born's brain, and thus would not be "you."

So, a head is all that is really needed. This still may strike some as macabre, and, as I say, it is somewhat controversial within the cryonics community. The controversy has to do with whether the essential " you" is all contained in your brain. Some feel our knowledge is insufficient to make such a claim. They think that there may be a form of identity memory in other parts of the body which might have to be linked to the brain in order for the essential "you" to be preserved.

On the other side of the controversy it is argued that people's personalities and memories seem to remain essentially the same in spite of loss of limbs, organ transplants, and paralysis resulting from high spinal cord injuries. Conversely, stroke victims, whose brain structures are damaged, do in fact lose memories and suffer personality changes. As long as the brain is undamaged, personality and memories appear to remain intact.

Obviously it is your choice as to which way you want to be suspended. Many people find the risk of a problem small and the savings large, and that probably explains the growing popularity of neurosuspension. At Alcor about 63% sign up for neurosuspensions and 27% for whole-body suspensions. Table 1 summarizes the pros and cons of whole-body versus neurosuspension.

Table 1. Whole-Body Vs. Neurosuspension

	ADVANTAGES	DISADVANTAGES
WHOLE-BODY SUSPENSION	Fully integrated organism to revive Will probably come out of suspension earlier More socially acceptable (as much as any of this is)	More costly to maintain More difficult to move in case of emergency
NEUROSUSPENSION (HEAD ONLY)	Less expensive to maintain Easier to move in case of emergency	Will probably come out of suspension later (more chance for culture shock) New body must be grown upon revival Chance that some form of memory will be lost Viewed as macabre by some

*Either way I might go, that's a big chunk of money that
I, for one, don't have, How do you expect an ordinary
person to take advantage of this even if they wanted to?
Or is this just for the rich?*

The most popular way to fund a suspension pro-
gram is through a life insurance policy. What happens is
that people take out a policy in the face amount they
need for the suspension and name the cryonics organization, such as Alcor, as the beneficiary of the policy.
The cryonics organization is thus assured of getting
their funds, assuming the person keeps up the premium
payments, when the person dies. That's not the only
way you can go, of course. If you happen to have a reasonably sizable estate, you can set up a trust fund benefiting the cryonics organization and accomplish the
same goal.

Either way the cryonics organization does not expect
to receive this money until after you have died and been
suspended. If such arrangements have not been made
ahead of time, however, the organization is not likely to
go through with the procedure. About 25%-50% of the
cost (depending on whether it is a whole-body or neuro
suspension) is incurred in carrying out the suspension
procedure. Thus, if the organization discovered after the
fact that no money would be forthcoming, they would
be out a substantial amount. The rest of the suspension
fee, beyond what is needed for the procedure itself, is
used primarily as interest bearing capital which will

cover maintenance costs indefinitely into the future until such time as you can be revived.

Table 2 will give you some idea of what it will cost to set up an insurance policy to cover your suspension. The premium amounts are for a non-smoking male and would result in a paid up policy after 20 years assuming an interest rate of 5 1/2%. The figures were provided by Roger Hartman and Company (see Resources section). Premiums would be less for a female and higher for a smoker.

Table 2. Monthly Premiums for Different Ages and Different Face Value Amounts

	FACE VALUE OF POLICY		
AGE	$30,000	$50,000	$120,000
20	$15	$22	$47
30	$20	$31	$71
40	$30	$48	$115
50	$50	$79	$190
60	$80	$128	$330

That seems a rather strange use of a life insurance policy.

On the contrary, what it means is that a life insurance policy is just that—*life* insurance, rather than what it normally is, *death* insurance. Ordinarily, you, personally, don't realize any gain from the face amount of your life insurance policy. Someone else gets the money when you die. A policy held for the purpose of preserving your body so that you can be brought back to life at some point in the future is in fact actually "insuring" your life.

Another way to think about it is that many religious people tithe their church, give a certain percentage of their earnings to the church. They do this partly in the hopes of gaining everlasting life. It's a different concept, a different scenario, but you could think of your insurance premiums as a tithing which has a very good chance of personally benefiting you.

How about the legality of this whole thing? What do I need to worry about there?

Legal matters fall into two broad categories, generic and personal. In the generic category lies the question of what the legal procedures are for carrying out a cryonic suspension. As mentioned earlier, current law requires that a person be declared legally dead before the suspension procedure can be initiated. This is not to the advantage of those on their deathbed wishing to be cryonically suspended. If death is sure, but the timing is not, it would obviously be very beneficial to be able to initiate the process at will. Alzheimers disease, for instance, destroys brain structure as do strokes. Preventing this damage will be important for the success of preserving the personality and the memories of the person suspended. The cryonic groups closely follow developments related to Dr. Jack Kevorkian's efforts and the assisted suicide movement as exemplified by Oregon's recently enacted law, but no significant changes in this area are likely for some time.

The problem can be especially aggravating for a person who does not reside close to a cryonics suspension center. You are about to die, but don't know when. If you have yourself transferred to the city where the suspension will take place, it could be a very expensive proposition waiting for legal death to occur while you are paying hotel or hospital bills. Conversely, it would also be very expensive for the cryonics organization to have a recovery team standing by indefinitely waiting for your legal death to take place, a situation which has in fact happened.

Another generic problem has to do with perpetuity laws. Since you are considered legally dead when you are suspended, there are complications arising from money set up in a trust fund in your name. After a certain number of years, which varies by state, the perpetuity laws will require dissolving the trust. Wisconsin is the only state which does not have such a law. One mechanism for getting around the perpetuity law and leaving money to yourself is to use a fund set up outside the United

States. For information on this option you should contact the Reanimation Foundation which has a fund set up in Liechtenstein (see Resources section). In any case, if you are interested in leaving money to yourself it would be best to consult an attorney.

There is also the question of the legal disposition of the body of a suspended person. The best current method of handling this seems to be for the body to be considered as an Anatomical Donation under the Uniform Anatomical Gift Act. The cryonics organization becomes the recipient of the gift. Make sure that your body parts are not donated to anyone other than your cryonics organization. They might make good use of them, but at your expense.

On the personal side, care must be taken in drawing up the legal documents which set up the disbursement of your assets, whether they are the proceeds from an insurance policy or a trust fund set up for the cryonics group. There are cases on record where surviving heirs have legally challenged the deceased's right to designate funds for cryonic suspension. (The challenges were unsuccessful.) You will also want to do what you can to make sure that either no autopsy is conducted on your body, or at the very least, that the autopsy be minimally invasive, particularly of the brain.

Once you are declared legally dead, you may or may not have any rights as an individual. In some states, California for instance, it has been established that the arrangements a person makes for the disposition of his or her body, such as for cryonic suspension, are valid. Obviously, it would be best to check the regulations in your state. If the state requires embalming (before the body can be air shipped) or an autopsy, your chances of a successful reanimation with all memories intact are significantly reduced. As cryonics becomes more popular and accepted, serious efforts should be made to change such laws and ensure the right of interested individuals to receive the best suspension possible. The best and most obvious change would be one which allowed the terminally ill to proceed with a suspension before the occurrence of legal death. Perhaps Dr. Jack Kevorkian's efforts will help lead to those sorts of change, as might the aforementioned "right to die" law in Oregon.

A recent article (Bridge, 1995) covers a number of legal issues concerning cryonics patients. Among other things it lists states where statutes have been passed allowing people to prevent autopsies based on "religious" objections. The statutes do not specify belief in any particular religion and the law has reportedly been used to prevent autopsies of two cryonics patients in California.

Cryonics organizations themselves are not immune from legal difficulties, as was well documented in a case involving the Alcor Foundation. In the Dora Kent case, the Riverside County coroner's office suspected foul play after her neurosuspension and wanted to perform an autopsy on the head after it had been frozen. Such an autopsy would have destroyed the very brain tissue the procedure was intended to preserve and ruined any chance for Dora Kent to be reanimated. After a lengthy court procedure with much expert testimony, Alcor prevailed and was able to maintain the integrity of Dora Kent's neuro-suspension. Alcor also had difficulty for a while in obtaining death certificates from the California State Health Department. The issue was resolved in court in Alcor's favor.

You might be interested in knowing the names of famous people who have been suspended or who have made suspension arrangements. So would I. But the cryonics organizations are very zealous, as they should be, in guarding the privacy of their members. Other than Dr. Timothy Leary, who has publicly announced the fact that he has made suspension arrangements, no other well known people have stepped forward. Then, of course, there's Elvis...no, no, no...let's not start another crazy rumor.

CHAPTER 18

Making Arrangements:
How To Ship Yourself
To the Future

> What the future has in store
> for you depends largely on
> what you place in store for
> the future.
>
> Evan Esar

In order for any of this to happen, you must have made arrangements to be cryonically suspended prior to being declared legally dead. This section of the book covers the details of how to make those arrangements. The cryonics organizations are listed under Resources at the end of the book.

There are three necessary kinds of arrangements you must make in order to be cryonically suspended. These include legal arrangements and financial arrangements. You also need to make the necessary arrangements so that the preliminary suspension process will begin as soon as possible after the moment of your legal death, and so that your body will then be transported to the place where the suspension will be completed.

Financial arrangements have already been discussed in the previous chapter under cost. As mentioned there, the most common method people use to pay for the suspension process is to name the cryonics organization as the beneficiary of an insurance policy. The other obvious method is to set up a trust fund with the cryonics organization as the beneficiary. Naturally, this requires that you have a large enough estate to cover at least the cost of a neurosuspension and that your trust be drawn up in such a way that it cannot be successfully contested by any heirs you may have. Other financial arrangements are possible, but need to be worked out on an individual basis with your cryonics organization.

When you sign up with the Alcor Foundation, you will receive an Application for Cryonic Suspension. (For information on the procedures used by other cryonics organizations listed in the Resource section, contact them.) The application covers the necessary legal matters and funding provisions and costs $150 to process. An administrator works closely with you to get the forms completed. Once you become a suspension member, there is an annual Emergency Responsibility Fee of $324. Your membership in Alcor yields a commitment on their part to have a recovery team standing by at your bedside if there is adequate warning that you are about to die, and if you live within a 100 mile radius of Phoenix. (You can make arrangements with Alcor for a standby recovery team outside the 100 mile radius by setting up a special fund.) The recovery team initiates the procedures described in Chapter 16 as soon as you are declared legally dead and transports your body to the suspension facility. If you die without warning, or you live further than 100 miles from Phoenix, the recovery team comes as soon as possible, but it will be crucial to have interim arrangements made to keep your body, in particular your head, cooled down to just above the freezing point of water. This delays the decay of the brain cells, which is the most important factor in this process. If at all possible, an anticoagulant, such as Heparin, should be injected.

If you know legal death is approaching, it will be important to pave the way in the best manner possible with whatever facility you are in, such as a hospital or a hospice. The desired outcome is that they relinquish custody of your body as quickly as possible to the recovery team. In a case where a recovery team is not used, your fate is completely in the hands of whomever you have designated to deal with the problem of getting your body transported to the suspension facility. The person might be your spouse, child, or friend. Of course, you must still have made arrangements with the cryonics organization to receive your body and perform the suspension procedure, but it will be up to your designated facilitator to get your body from the place of legal death to the cryonic suspension facility. Crude but effective methods for improving your chances of successful reanimation include packing the body immediately in ice to cool it down as much as possible and shipping it with an adequate supply of ice to keep it cooled until it reaches its destination. The cryonics organizations can provide more detailed information in this area. Alcor, for instance, reports that morticians often prove cooperative and can help with the necessary procedures.

So, it sounds as if my best bet is to live in the same city as the cryonics group I belong to?

It is your best bet, but this may be the place to start thinking about a necessary balance in your life. I view the situation as comparable to the issue of saving money for your retirement. There is a tightrope, of sorts, one has to walk. If you put your total focus on the future, on retirement, you will deny yourself many of the pleasures of the present. Don't buy a new car, wear old clothes, never take an expensive vacation, etc.. If you happen to die before retirement age you will have had the dubious pleasure of having denied yourself almost all of life's pleasures in order to leave a nice nest egg for your heirs.

However, if you live for the moment with no thought for your financial needs down the road, and live to be one hundred and twenty, you may find yourself in an equally dismal situation. Plenty of time and no wherewithal with which to enjoy it.

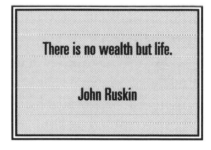

There is no wealth but life.

John Ruskin

Cryonics is much the same. Keep in mind that cryonic suspension is not a sure thing (we'll talk in a later chapter about the kinds of things that may go wrong). Rearranging your life and priorities just to maximize the chances of receiving a "good" suspension may deprive you of some worthwhile pleasures in your current life— foreign travel, for instance. But, ignoring the whole topic would not seem wise either. There are some steps you can take, one being to make sure others in your environment know about your wishes and the arrangements you have made. Cryonics organizations typically provide something to carry on your person, such as a bracelet, necklace, or card which will let others know whom to contact in case of your actual or imminent death. Such measures won't interfere much with your enjoyment of the moment, but will enhance your suspension chances. Again, a balance of concerns seems to make the most sense here.

A new type of community is being contemplated for those who want to improve their odds and who are willing to move to do so. The Venturist organization (see Resources) is hoping to set up a retirement community in Scottsdale which would include a hospice for those who will soon need suspension. The hospice would include monitoring devices in case a patient died in the middle of the night and would obviously be conducive to beginning suspensions promptly.

The only other kind of arrangement you might want to think about making would be to make funds available for your personal use upon being reanimated, whenever that may be. A natural thought would be that you simply set aside some money for yourself, put it in the care of the trust department of some stable bank, and assume that you're going to wake up with a very sizable nest egg, depending on how long it takes before you are reanimated. Unfortunately, as already mentioned, the perpetuity laws in all but one state currently prohibit such an arrangement. Once you are legally dead you cannot have a trust fund benefiting you which lasts longer than a certain number of years. As discussed earlier, one option would be to invest your funds someplace where there is no perpetuity law such as in the Reanimation Foundation (see Resources section). Depending on how long your funds sit accruing interest, waiting for you to reappear, you could build up a very nice amount. And, again, consulting your lawyer about such matters is a good idea.

CHAPTER 19

The Mental Obstacle Course: Part Two

> A great deal of money is expended on funerals and that, in itself, seems to betray a lack of confidence in the resurrection of the dead.
>
> Dr. Edward Henderson

What's the matter with you anyway? Afraid of getting old and dying?

Well, yes, actually. Let's face it, for very good reasons humans have made a virtue out of a necessity when it comes to the topics of aging and dying. Aging gracefully, the slow accretion of wisdom, living life to the fullest (for tomorrow we die), mature acceptance of one's mortal fate—all of these abilities and attitudes are, in general, admired by society.

Worrying obsessively about dying, or the counterpart, refusing to talk about it or deal with it, is not an admirable trait. Good arguments can be made that society values the traits appropriately when death is the certain outcome of life. But what if death is not certain? If death is not a sure thing, should we admire someone who accepts it? I wouldn't. In a similar vein, does society currently give its approbation to those who commit suicide? Generally not. It could be argued that not taking a chance on prolonging your life indefinitely through cryonic suspension is a form of suicide. There are many ways to kill yourself. Failing to take the steps necessary to keep yourself alive is one such way. So how is suicide different from ignoring cryonics? Yeah, OK, it's cheaper, but other than that?

Often the test of courage is not to die but to live.

Vittorio Alfieri

Those who view death as always and forever certain will have a much different view of cryonics from those holding the opposite opinion. One man's foolish desperation will be another's well-calculated and reasonable gamble. And, as with politics and religion, arguing about the matter probably won't change many opinions. So if you choose to arrange for suspension, and tell others about it, you will have to be prepared to be considered odd at best and perhaps death obsessed (when in reality you are life obsessed). But "he who laughs last laughs best" was never more appropriate as a consoling thought.

One would expect that if fear of death was the main motivating force for people to sign up for suspension, those signing up would primarily be the old. In fact, most arranging to be suspended are of the baby-boomer generation, not the elderly. This suggests that faith in technology may be a more important motivating factor than fear of dying. In any case, cryonicists are people with a strong desire to live, not die.

> Do not go gentle into that good night,
> Old age should burn and rave at close of day;
> Rage, rage against the dying of the light.
>
> Dylan Thomas

I've got family and I wonder if this isn't somehow cheating them. I mean if I take out a life insurance policy and they don't get the proceeds, or if I take something out of my will... Is that something I can really feel good about?

The whole issue of family and loved ones can be a very complex and emotion-wrought area. I think a starting point is to make sure that none of this comes as a surprise to anyone close to you. It should be discussed with them, and they should have knowledge of what your wishes are, in part just to make sure that your wishes are carried out. They should also know ahead of time so that at a traumatic moment, when medical science can no longer keep you alive, you don't add another level to their trauma. Finding out at the last moment that you've made plans to be suspended rather than having your body disposed of in more traditional fashion could be a considerable shock, especially if you've chosen the neurosuspension option.

I would suggest that the occasion on which you announce your intentions to your family and loved ones be a fairly formal one, one which you've spent some time thinking through. It's a big decision which might be viewed by some as selfish, especially in light of fact that you are diverting some of your resources to cryonic suspension. These are resources which otherwise some members of your family could expect to receive. Also, the topic of death is emotional, and not one people like to contemplate and discuss.

The thrust of the conversation from your point of view can be that you have hopeful news. You are not necessarily trying to convince them to go the same route you're going, but you view your decision to be cryonically suspended as a very positive, life-affirming one. You don't consider the end of your current life as the ultimate end. You have hope for the future which you want to share with them.

There is no getting around the fact that what you're doing is likely be seen by some as selfish. Assume, though, that you were lying on your near-death bed with a fatal disease and were offered the opportunity to have an expensive new treatment that seemed to hold good promise of curing you. Further assume that your medical insurance did not cover the procedure. Would your loved ones begrudge you using whatever resources you had available to pay for the treatment? Would they see that as within your purview?

I believe that in most cases family would think that it would be legitimate to use your own resources to try to prolong your life. The difference between selling your house (or using your life savings) to get an experimental new medical treatment and using some portion of your assets to be cryonically suspended is quite simple. In one case use of your resources will perhaps extend your life by a few months or years at best. In the case of cryonic suspension, use of those funds may extend your life indefinitely. It seems that if there is any difference between those two kinds of uses of your funds, it clearly favors cryonic suspension. Being suspended is no more, or less, selfish than selling your house to pay for some experimental medical treatment.

> *OK, but suppose I spend that money and get cheated? Why would anybody bother to reanimate me even if they could?*

Your question assumes that the capability to reanimate you exists but that it is not used for some reason. We'll speak in the next chapter about natural disasters and other inadvertent reasons why you might not get reanimated. The topic for now is willful neglect, either by your cryonic organization or as imposed by society. Let's deal first with the cryonic organization.

Given that the organization had the technological capability and financial resources to reanimate you, what reason would they have for refusing to do so? When you sign up with one of these organizations you are entering into a legal agreement whereby you agree to provide funds and they agree to suspend and then reanimate you when it becomes possible. There is plenty of evidence of ineptness among the early cryonics organizations, but, with one possible exception, none of fraud. Four of the organizations currently in existence have been around for a number of years and are composed primarily of people who will someday be suspended themselves and are consequently depending for their revival on those who follow

them. Although one of the first people involved in cryonics had a profit motive (Perry, 1993), it has not proven
to be a fertile area for those hoping to make a fast buck.
That could change in the future as its popularity rises, of
course, but there is little reason now to believe that any
cryonics organization, given the capability, would will-
fully fail to revive a suspended person under their care.

Turning now to society, what reasons could exist
which would cause society to intervene and not allow
the cryonics organizations to revive their suspended
patients? Remember, we are assuming the capability to
reanimate and the willingness of the cryonics organizations to perform. Why would society not allow reanimation? The most likely reason would have to do with overpopulation and limited resources. As we've already
discussed, the technology necessary for reanimation,
nanotechnology, will make us capable of supporting a
much larger population on Earth and also capable of
expanding into space. It is doubtful, given present
trends, that the number of people suspended will ever be
a very large percentage of the population.

Given the pace at which technology changes, as con-
trasted to the pace at which most people understand and
accept those changes, nanotechnology will probably be
developed before most people accept cryonics. Even if
cryonic suspension became wildly more popular than it
is now and there were a million patients waiting to be
reanimated, they would still represent an extremely small
percentage of the world population. Adding such a small

percentage to the overall population is unlikely to unduly strain resources and could be accomplished in a phased fashion to minimize whatever strain it did cause.

The other likely reason for a societal prohibition of reanimations would probably be based on some religious or philosophical considerations. Such things are difficult to predict from our present position, but highlight an area of concern for those interested in cryonics. That concern has to do with the legal status of suspended patients. Since they are legally dead, it might be difficult to protect their rights if a law should be passed forbidding their reanimation. Of course there is a precedent for following the wishes of someone legally dead. We do honor the wills of the dead and generally carry out their wishes concerning the disposition of the body. Probably the best one can do for now is to hope for the continuation of our open, democratic, society with its well established respect for life and individual rights. It may be that as cryonics continues to grow in popularity it will be possible to bring a favorable resolution to the question of legal status and rights for those suspended.

> **It is better to be a mouse in a cat's mouth than to be a man in a lawyer's hands.**
>
> **Spanish Proverb**

CHAPTER 20

Dealing with Murphy's Law: Preventing What Might Go Wrong

> Man blames fate for other accidents, but feels personally responsible when he makes a hole in one.
>
> Horizons Magazine

In an uncertain world nothing is for sure, and that easily includes being successfully reawakened from a cryonic suspension. So let's talk about various possibilities for what might go wrong and whether there are any steps that you can take to minimize the chances of a problem for you. We'll start at the far end of the time stream and work our way back.

The obvious possibility at the far end of the time stream is that the technology is never developed which would make it possible to bring you back to life from your cryonic suspension. This would mean that nanotechnology is never developed to the stage of cellular repair and that no other technology is developed which would make cellular repair possible.

We discussed earlier the kinds of catastrophic global events which might prevent the development of nanotechnology. Short of those kinds of catastrophes, or of a complete collapse of scientific and technological advance by the human race, nanotechnology or some other technology capable of cellular repair would seem to be nearly inevitable, as argued in Chapter 5. Clearly, though, this is one area where things could go wrong with the consequence that you never awaken to your dream of the future. It is also true that there is little you can do to affect this potential problem other than pushing the nanotechnology cause while you're still around.

Another possible way that things can go wrong for you is that the cellular repair capability of nanotechnology *does* get developed, but for some reason it is not used to revive you. There are two categories of possibilities here. One possibility is that no one gets revived. The other possibility is that some people get revived, but you don't.

No One Gets Revived

One probable cause could be the cost of the procedure. As explained earlier, however, nanotechnology should be very inexpensive, including the sophisticated level of technology necessary to reanimate cryonically suspended patients.

There could also be some legal or societal prohibition which prevents the reanimation of anyone, even though it has become technically possible. Once you are suspended, of course, there is little you can do—OK, make that *nothing* you can do—to change such prohibitions. Working toward acceptance of nanotechnology and cryonics *now* could have an important impact on your future prospects.

Another possibility is that nanotechnology can indeed reanimate your body, but the hypothesis about the structural nature of memory is wrong, and the "you" that is the sum of your memories has vanished. As Chapter 12 states, however, the growing consensus of research does support the hypothesis that the physical structure contains your memory. If memory is encoded in the positioning of atoms and molecules in your brain, and if those atoms and molecules are still in place when the nanomachines begin coursing through your suspended body, then you and your memories should be safe.

In Chapter 4 I touched on the matter of the "soul" long enough to suggest that it was not a concern of this technological, practical book. Now that the basic ideas of the book have been presented, we should perhaps briefly revisit the topic, because some might argue that whether or not anyone will be revived is dependent on just what happens to the soul during cryonic suspension.

If one believes in a soul there are two logical possibilities, either the soul departs when one is cryonically suspended or it doesn't. If it doesn't, it will still be there when the person is revived and there is no problem. If the soul departs, it could either be gone permanently or come back when the person was revived. If it comes back, there is again no problem. If the soul departs permanently, however, when does it go and why? These seem to me unanswerable questions. The only guidance we have from previous experience is that people who would once have been declared legally dead have been brought back to life and seem to suffer no ill effects. Did they lose their souls? Science has no answers for such metaphysical questions.

Others Get Revived, You Don't

Suppose it's just you, or some sub-group of people including you, not getting revived. One possible cause could be the failure of the cryonics organization which suspended you to carry out its reanimation obligation when the technology becomes available. The most likely reason for this failure would be that the organization lacks the financial resources to complete its obligations.

Clearly, it is to your advantage to choose your cryonics organization with an eye towards organizational and financial stability and to strongly support the one you choose.

Marching back in time, another possibility for where things might go wrong is that some compromise of the storage facility or the tank in which your body is contained occurs, causing you to prematurely thaw. This could be caused by natural or man-made disasters or by some failure of the cryonics organization. The threat of earthquakes was a primary factor in Alcor's decision to recently move their facility from southern California to Scottsdale, Arizona. There is, however, little organizations or individuals can do about the possibility of other kinds of devastating disasters such as war and civil unrest.

The negative consequences of organizational failure again point to the necessity of choosing a cryonics organization which gives the highest quality of care to suspended patients and has the best chance of surviving as an organization. Although a suspended patient does not need much care, the small amount needed is crucial.

In this respect, it is comforting to know that storage in liquid nitrogen is not dependent on an uninterrupted supply of electricity. As long as the tanks are topped up with liquid nitrogen every eight to ten days storage remains secure. Of course a major catastrophe which paralyzes the storage city for a sustained period of time could threaten the organization's ability to maintain its suspended patients because of lack of personnel or resupply capability. It is important to note here that there is almost a family feeling among the cryonics organizations, albeit families which squabble with one another. A person on duty during a disturbance of some sort is not likely to view what he or she is doing as just a job, and drop all responsibilities at the first sign of trouble. Most of the people working in a cryonics facility expect to be suspended themselves someday and know that they will be dependent on the care of those that follow them for their own survival through the suspension period.

Working our way back in time, we come to potential problems with the suspension process itself. The most basic of these potential problems would be that somehow the steps taken during the suspension are not sufficient to preserve your memories and personality, meaning that only your physical body will be revived. The cryonics organizations are doing what they can to support research on improved methods of suspension, but there is good reason to hope that current methods are sufficient. The evidence cited earlier on the structural nature of memory, the fact that these structures are not irreparably harmed by freezing, and the step-by-step revival scenario given by Fahy are all persuasive reasons for such hope. The suspension process itself, of course, is a surgical procedure, and we all know that things can go wrong during surgery. Problems during suspension which compromise the brain structures are the most serious possibility. Supporting the research on suspension procedures, if you can, and choosing an experienced cryonics organization are the best preventative steps you can take for this category of potential problems.

The next area of concern has to do with what happens to your body in between the time of legal death and the time you reach the suspension facility. Basically, what can go wrong here is that too long a time-lapse will occur between legal death and the suspension process being started. If that happens, the inevitable decay of brain structure will destroy too much of your memories for the real you to be revived. Obviously, that delay could occur in various ways.

There could be trouble in the transportation, some problem with the response team, or problems getting your body released by a hospital or hospice. You might die in a foreign country where it would take too long for your body to get cooled down or sent back to the suspension facility. You might die alone in some place where your body is not found for some time.

This sounds like a real likely place for things to go wrong. How long do I have before it's too late?

Since the important thing is the preservation of the structures of the brain, the key question is how long it takes before structural integrity is lost. There is a very common misconception that the brain is irreparably harmed after about 4 or 5 minutes of oxygen deprivation (see Smith 1989, p.118, for instance). In fact, what happens is that the brain cell *processes* often cannot be restarted with current technology after that period of time. The *structures* of the brain, however, remain intact for several hours after the heart stops (Drexler, 1986, pp. 266-267). Furthermore, "...individual brain cells...preserve their ability to synthesize RNA for more than five hours after cessation of general circulation..." (Zakharova and Tumanov, 1992). Thus, even brain processes which we cannot currently restart continue for hours after death.

So, how likely is it that your suspension process will start before any structural damage to the brain begins? That depends in part on the preparations you've made, in part on lifestyle, and in part on luck. Preparations include notifying those in your environment about what needs to be done in case of your deanimation and carrying some sort of identification, such as a necklace, card, or bracelet to notify strangers of your wishes in case you can't. Lifestyle issues include the question of whether you live alone or with others, how much travelling you do, and whether you engage in risky behaviors which might cause you to die alone and out of the notice of others. Such behaviors would include skiing in remote locations, hunting alone, etc.. Another life style issue concerns how many others committed to cryonics live in your area. Clearly, the larger the support group the better your chances. You can either increase this number by moving to a location where there is a nucleus of such people, Scottsdale Arizona for instance, or by getting others in your area interested.

If it weren't for bad luck I wouldn't have any luck at all.

Unknown

No one can control Lady Luck, but there are some statistics which are comforting. More than 70% of all deaths in the United States and Britain are "negotiated" as to their time (Death: The Trip of a Lifetime, PBS, 1993). This means that someone decides that a dying patient should have "the plug pulled," i.e., that artificial means, such as heart and lung machines, of keeping the patient alive should be discontinued. Conversely, this means that fewer than 30% of all people in the US and Great Britain die under uncontrolled circumstances. Alcor reports that 26% of those they have suspended died unexpectedly (Cryonics, 1993, p.37). It is these uncontrolled deaths which are the ones most likely to lead to delayed suspension procedures. In fact, the figure is probably lower than 30% because many in that 30% which are not negotiated as to time of death no doubt still expire in a hospital or a hospice setting. Any deaths in such settings increase the probability of timely and successful suspensions.

Of course dying in a hospital gives no assurance that suspension can be started immediately. It depends very much on the attitudes and cooperation of the attending physician and the hospital. Although Alcor reports generally good cooperation, there have been instances when suspensions have been delayed by physicians and hospital administrators.

> "Because cryonics is currently deemed to be outside the purview of medicine, the general problem is most often the failure of the physician, hospital, and/or other related authorities to cooperate with (or simply *not interfere with*) the cryonics organization in the event of an emergency." (Cryonics, 1993 p.30).

The solution to these kinds of problems will come eventually as cryonics and the associated enabling technologies become known and accepted. The best you can do at present is to make sure that your doctor and your hospital know in advance what your wishes are and that you try to deal with any complications before the fact. Meantime, Alcor reports that problems of this nature have only delayed, not prevented, past suspensions.

Chapter 21

Decisions, Decisions

> Take calculated risks.
> That is quite different
> from being rash.
>
> George S. Patton

As you will have surmised by now, nothing is certain in any of this. What we are dealing with are trends and probabilities—technological trends and a number of probabilities relating to your chances of benefiting from those trends. Although we haven't spoken much about values, the implicit assumption of the book is that you, the reader, would place a positive value on perfect health, youth, and immortality. That may be wrong, but

I suspect that if it's vastly wrong you wouldn't be reading this book.

Now that all the basic elements of the book have been covered, it might be time to step back and to try to put everything into a coherent picture. The picture will help you make a decision—and of course you *will* be making a decision about what to do with the information in this book, one way or the other. Once you complete the book, the first basic decision is either to do something based on what you've read or not. Closing the book and then dismissing it from your mind *is* a decision. So how would you go about deciding whether or not to do any-thing?

Warning to those with math phobia. The formal decision model presented in the next section uses numbers and a simple formula. If your eyes begin to glaze, just skip ahead to the section labeled "Informal Decisions".

Formal Decision Model

People use all sorts of methods to make decisions, most of them pretty informal. My suggestion, since this is a major decision, is that you use a formal method. Much of the value of using a well thought-out decision process is that it helps you uncover the most important elements of the decision. As an example to get you started, we'll look at one fairly simple decision analysis model called Subjective Expected Utility. It may sound a little formidable, but it's really a pretty straightforward concept as you'll see. We'll look at the model first and then explain the terms used. The model says that the Subjective Expected Utility (SEU) of some choice is simply the product of the subjective probability of the outcome multiplied by the utility of that outcome, or

SEU = subjective probability x utility

According to the model there are really only two subjective elements to any decision. One has to do with your estimate of the probability that something will happen. The "something happens" we'll call an "outcome." Since the important thing is *your* estimate of the probability of the outcome, we'll call it "subjective probability." For instance, the objective probability that something might happen will not be the salient feature for you if the objective probability differs significantly from your subjective opinion. If you are afraid of flying, for instance, the objective probability that you will die in a plane crash will likely be much different from your subjective probability. All the talk in the world about how much more dangerous automobiles are will have little effect on your level of terror as the plane rumbles down the runway.

The other subjective quantity has to do with the value you place on that something happening, that outcome. Since, again, the important thing is *your* estimate of the value of the outcome, we'll call the value "utility" to indicate that it also is a subjective quantity. For instance, a hundred dollars might be the "value" of some object, but its "utility" to you could be more or less than that. On the one hand, if it's a case of shark repellent and you are dying of thirst in the desert, it won't be worth anything to you. On the other hand, if you are in a raft on the ocean being attacked by a school of sharks, a case of shark repellent might have a utility of far more than a hundred dollars.

OK, I see the point, but what does all this have to do with immortality?

My suggestion is that you use the Subjective Expected Utility model to help you decide what to do with your new-found knowledge about nanotechnology, cryonics, and your chance to become immortal. At this point there are two basic alternatives you can choose between. One alternative is to make arrangements to be cryonically suspended, and the other is to not do that. Likewise, there are two states the world might evolve to over the relevant period of time. In one state people who are cryonically suspended are revived into a beneficial new world. In the other state they are not revived. (For the sake of simplicity we will ignore the chance that you might survive to the era of nanotechnology cell repair without being suspended.)

So we now we have a little 2X2 table that looks like Table 3 and we can fill in the outcomes, which are the cells.

Table 3. SEU Model For Cryonic Suspension Decision

		STATE OF THE WORLD	
		1. REVIVAL	2. NO REVIVAL
A C T I O N	A. SUSPENSION		
	B. NO SUSPENSION		

The cells represent combinations of actions chosen (to be suspended or not) and future world states (suspendees revived or not). If you choose to become suspended and the future state of the world is one where you can be revived, then the outcome is immortality. If you choose to be suspended but the world does not turn out to be in the state where you get revived, then the outcome is death.

If you choose not to be suspended and people can be

Table 4.
SEU Model for Cryonic Suspension Decision: Outcomes

		STATE OF THE WORLD	
		1. REVIVAL	2. NO REVIVAL
A C T I O N	A. SUSPENSION	OUTCOME 1A: IMMORTALITY	OUTCOME 2A: DEATH
	B. NO SUSPENSION	OUTCOME 1B: DEATH	OUTCOME 2B: DEATH

revived, the outcome of course is death. If you choose not to be suspended and no one is revived, then your outcome is still death. So one way of looking at this is that you have one chance at immortality. Table 4 shows the outcomes filled in.

There is more involved, however, so let's break the problem down a little further. The first step is to assign some probabilities to the two future world states. Just for the sake of illustration let's say that your current subjective probability that people will be revived is 50%. That means you would assess a 50% probability for that state and a 50% probability for the state in which nobody is revived. The 50% probability is an estimate which covers a whole host of elements having probabilities attached to them. It includes, for instance, that cellular repair nanotechnology is developed, that nothing goes wrong with your suspension process or with the organization storing your body, etc.

> **Long-range planning does not deal with future decisions, but with the future of present decisions.**
>
> **Peter Drucker**

You'll have a chance a little later to plug in different probabilities if you want. For now, the next question is—what value do these various outcomes have for you? This gets a little more complicated, but let's assume your utility for outcomes ranges along a scale from -100 to +100, with -100 being the worst and +100 being the best. The first question then is what utility would you assign to the outcome where you chose to be suspended and you do get revived (Outcome 1A)? Let's assume that would be the highest utility (as it would be for me), and assign it a value of +100.

Now, what would be the utility for you if you choose to be suspended, it doesn't work, and legal death becomes memory death (Outcome 2A)? When I think about the utility of this outcome, I have to include the cost, both psychic and monetary, associated with choosing to become suspended. We've talked about the psychic costs of friends and family thinking that you're a kook. Obviously, there is some sacrifice involved in paying for insurance premiums if you don't have a sizeable enough estate set up a trust fund. On the positive side, I like the thought of being associated with a cutting-edge venture on the frontier of science, even if it ultimately doesn't work out for me personally. All of those positive and negative factors go into this outcome, and it winds up, for me, with a negative utility. I made all those sacrifices, and I get almost nothing for it. Of course, since I'll be dead I won't know that, but we're trying to make the decision now. So I'm going to say that for me this has a utility of -30, and I'll assume it is the same for you.

Now to the next scenario, represented by the bottom two cells. The utility for me of choosing not to be suspended when I could have awakened in a world full of immortals (Outcome 1B) is the most negative outcome possible, so that gets a -100. And, if I choose not to do it and if in fact it wouldn't have worked anyway (Outcome 2B), I have a positive utility. I made the right decision, I didn't squander my time and resources, and I took no psychic beating from friends and family. In fact no matter what I did, I was doomed to die, and that's what happened. It's not as good an outcome for me as becoming immortal, so I'm not going to assign it a +100, but I'll say it's worth +50. Table 5 shows the probabilities and utilities filled in.

Table 5. SEU Model For Cryonic Suspension Decision: Outcomes, Probabilities and Utilities

		STATE OF THE WORLD	
		1. REVIVAL PROBABILITY = .50	2. NO REVIVAL PROBABILITY = .50
A C T I O N	A. SUSPENSION	OUTCOME 1: IMMORTALITY UTILITY = +100	OUTCOME 2A: DEATH UTILITY = -30
	B. NO SUSPENSION	OUTCOME 2B: DEATH UTILITY = -100	OUTCOME 2B: DEATH UTILITY = +50

We're now in a position to figure out the Subjective Expected Utility for each action. What this represents is simply your feeling about what the outcomes are worth to you weighted by how probable you think they are. The calculation will allow us to see which course of action is likely to give you a higher expected utility. To do that we just take the probability of the world states and multiply them by the utilities of the outcomes. Then we add them together for each possible action, or decision alternative.

Subjective Expected Utility of **Suspension**

For the alternative of choosing to be suspended we've got .50 probability times a utility of +100 plus .50 probability times a utility of -30. Fully worked out, it looks like this:

SEU=(Prob. of revival x Utility of 1A) + (Prob. of no revival x Utility of 2A)

SEU = (.5 x 100) + (.5 x -30)
SEU = (50) + (-15)
SEU = 35

For the alternative of choosing not to be suspended we have:

Subjective Expected Utility of **No suspension**

SEU=(Prob. of revival x Utility of 1B) + (Prob. of no revival x Utility of 2B)

SEU = (.5 x -100) + (.5 x 50)
SEU = (-50) + (25)
SEU = -25

Most people would rather die than think: many do.
Bertrand Russell

Since I used my own subjective probabilities and utilities in the example, you can see that my SEU is highest for choosing to be suspended. In fact, I have made arrangements to be suspended. Now, how about you? All you need to do is put in your own estimates of the probabilities and your own utilities associated with each outcome and what it takes to get you to that outcome. You'll find that Table 6 and the following SEU

Table 6. Blank SEU Model For Cryonic Suspension Decision: Outcomes, Probabilities and Utilities

		STATE OF THE WORLD	
		1. REVIVAL PROBABILITY =	2. NO REVIVAL PROBABILITY =
A C T I O N	A. SUSPENSION	OUTCOME 1A: IMMORTALITY UTILITY =	OUTCOME 2A: DEATH UTILITY =
	B. NO SUSPENSION	OUTCOME 1B: DEATH UTILITY =	OUTCOME 2B: DEATH UTILITY =

equations are blank and waiting for you to jot in your own numbers and do the arithmetic if you so desire.

Subjective Expected Utility of **Suspension**

SEU=(Prob. of revival x Utility of 1A) + (Prob. of no revival x Utility of 2A)

SEU =

Subjective Expected Utility of **No suspension**

SEU=(Prob. of revival x Utility of 1B) + (Prob. of no revival x Utility of 2B)

SEU =

Ralph Merkle in a recent article (1993) makes an interesting observation having to do with the subjective probability part of the equation. He observes that as knowledge of nanotechnology and its capabilities spread, it will undoubtedly have an effect on the subjective probability people associate with successful reanimation. As more and more people reach their decision threshold for being suspended (although Merkle's threshold is for a probability, not a Subjective Expected Utility), more and more will do so.

An increased probability for successful revivals obviously also increases the Subjective Expected Utility for choosing to be suspended, and should also move people over the threshold. Of course, both observations assume that people make these kinds of decisions in some rational manner. You do, don't you? Note that the numbers (probabilities and utilities) are subject to change over time. You might decide that making arrangements to become suspended is not the optimal decision this year. Changes in your utilities, or advances in technology which affect the probability of revival, may reverse that judgment at a later date. One final thought. If there is any chance you might change your mind later, it would make good sense to take out the additional insurance needed now, while your rates are as low as they're going to get.

Informal Decisions

Perhaps numbers and rational decision models are not your cup of tea. You could think of your decision as a complaint reduction mechanism. (If you're perfectly satisfied with your life and never complain, you can skip this section—and please send me your secret.) Have you ever wished you had trained for a different career, had a healthier body, could travel more, had more time to enjoy yourself, or____ (fill in your favorite complaint or wish)? In the world of the future you'll have a chance to fix those problems, realize those dreams. All you need to do is get there. Choose to live, not to die.

Let's look at your decision from yet another point of view, that of regret. Though their names are not known, there are a group of people who are of historical importance for being the last of their kind. Who, for instance, was the last person to die of smallpox? This disease has now been eradicated and the smallpox virus exists only in a safeguarded laboratory. Someone had the distinction of being its last victim. Diphtheria which used to cause 15,000 deaths a year in the United States has almost been eradicated (FDA Consumer, 1990). Polio has been eliminated in the Western Hemisphere. It is predicted that a cure for cystic fibrosis will be available within the next ten to fifteen years.

Because of poverty and lack of medical care there are still people dying from diseases which could easily have been prevented. From the point of view of inevitability, these people are dying needlessly. But, one can optimistically assume that in the not too distant future adequate medical care will be available to everyone. Someone now alive, for instance, could well be the last person to die of a pneumonia which could have been cured with a simple antibiotic.

Now, imagine that you were a person dying of pneumonia before the discovery of penicillin and all the other antibiotics. Further imagine that someone offered to put you to sleep until a cure could be found for your pneumonia. Would you have accepted that offer? Would you have accepted life? If the promise of cellular repair nanotechnology is fulfilled, there will someday be a person who is the *last* to die with no chance of being resurrected in a new body with all memories intact. Given the current lack of popularity of cryonics and the current lack of knowledge about the potential of nanotechnology, undoubtedly billions are yet doomed to die. Now that you have the knowledge imparted by this book, you could be among the first to avoid a dubious distinction...the distinction of having died just before the dawning of the era of immortality. Decisions, decisions.

> To do nothing is in every man's power.
>
> Samuel Johnson

THE
WORLD
OF YOUR
FUTURE

CHAPTER 22

Paradise Enough: From Star Travel To "Smart" Clothes

> My interest is in the future because I am going to spend the rest of my life there.
>
> Charles F. Kettering

OK, say I do it, I go into suspension. What kind of a world am I likely to wake up in?

As I said before, making precise predictions about the future is a fool's game. There are several givens implied in your question, though, which make it possible to paint some broad brush strokes. First, we can assume that you have awakened from your suspension. Thus we can be assured that nanotechnology, or some equally powerful but as yet unknown technology, has made it possible to repair the freezing damage to your body, and to repair the problems that led to your suspension. So, the world in which you wake will have those powers, and they in turn mean the existence of the other capabilities of nanotechnology.

We've talked in general terms about those capabilities and the benefits they will bring. Those benefits range from cheaply produced goods, to perfect health, to no aging, to cheap transportation, and cheap spaceflight. Now let's try to fill out the picture somewhat. Because cellular repair nanotechnology represents one of the most sophisticated, advanced versions of nanotechnology, we can be assured that not only will nanotechnology be available when you awaken but that the world will also have had the benefits of the technology for some time. Thus we will be examining a fairly mature nanotechnology society. The topics chosen for the following discussion are illustrative and are meant to give some idea of the scope of the changes which can be expected.

The future is hidden even from the men who make it.

Anatole France

As likely details of the future world are discussed, keep in mind that nanotechnology will bring fundamental changes in the way we live, just as the inventions of agriculture, industrial machines, and information technology did. Imagine trying to explain to a peasant of the middle ages all the changes in day-to-day living which would take place as a consequence of the industrial revolution. Most of the major elements would have sounded fantastic and implausible in the extreme. So, keep that mind of yours propped open. We'll begin with the stars and work our way down to the clothing against your skin.

Star Travel

One of the immutable laws of nature has to do with the maximum speed with which we can travel. We are limited to traveling at the speed of light, and even that is only a theoretical limit to be approached but never reached. Since the nearest star system to Earth is over four light years away, this means it would take a minimum of four years travel to reach that star system and another four years to return to Earth. At half the speed of light the trip would take eight years each way. To reach an interesting star system with habitable planets might take very much longer, depending on where the nearest one is located. Such lapses of time seem quite daunting in our present age, even if we had the space hardware and support systems to allow a human to remain in space that long and reach those distant goals.

Further compounding the time-lapse problem is that as a space ship approaches an appreciable fraction of the speed of light, time on board the ship runs at a different rate. More time will pass on Earth than on the ship, and the faster the ship goes the greater will be the differential. This unlikely sounding effect follows directly from Einstein's Theory of General Relativity. Friends and family you leave behind on Earth could grow old and die before you return still in the prime of your life.

In an era of nanotechnology things will be quite different. Three factors will strongly affect the feasibility of interstellar travel. These factors are the cost of transportation, control over our bodies, and the importance of the passage of time. We'll start with the last one first.

As mentioned above, one of the consequences of traveling at near-light speeds has to do with relativistic effects on time. Essentially, the faster you and your spacecraft travel the more time slows down for you (as seen from the perspective of an observer on Earth). If you traveled to Alpha Centauri (about four light years away) and back, at half the speed of light you'd be over two years younger than you'd have been if you stayed on Earth. If you travel longer distances or at higher fractions of the speed of light, the time disparity increases. While a year is passing for you, twenty-five years may be passing for those you left behind on Earth.

In our current era, these sorts of relativistic time shifts can be discouraging. In terms of people you know and love and the world as you know it, you are essentially going on a one way mission if you take a very long interstellar trip. So many years will have passed on Earth before you return that no one you knew will be left alive and the world may be vastly different. In an age of immortals, where life spans are indefinitely long, this should not be as big a consideration. The same large chunks of time will pass for the people you are close to and their lives will have gone on, but they will still be around when you get back.

Travel to the stars will also be made feasible by the cheap manufacturing costs associated with nanotechnology. Much of the design for an interstellar ship would be accomplished through automated systems engineering. The ship "seed" containing all of the information needed to build the ship and some nanomachine assemblers could be placed in an environment rich in the needed materials (such as the asteroid belt). With very little human intervention, a mighty starship could be built. The nanoassemblers and nanocomputers would build the molecular and macro-level machines necessary to mine and transport raw materials, process the materials, and turn them into a finished product of great complexity.

One current idea for motive power for such a star ship is to use solar sails pushed by laser beams generated in solar orbit. As the star ship approaches its destination, it is decelerated by a laser built by nanoseeds sent on earlier. Such a ship would be relatively slow, operating only at a fraction of the speed of light, but other more advanced designs are at least in the conceptual stage.

With the advent of nanotechnology, many other possible avenues for power will likely become available.

A serious problem for interstellar travelers, given what we know currently, has to do with the effects of prolonged exposure of the human body to the conditions of space. The absence of gravity seems to have a fairly rapid diminishing effect on bone mass and could lead to debilitation after a much shorter period of time than it would take to reach even the nearer stars. The brute force mechanical answer to that problem would be to rotate the star ship in such a fashion that artificial gravity is produced. A more sophisticated possibility, based on the capabilities of nanotechnology, would simply be to maintain the body through cellular repair nanomachines. Thus the debilitating effects of weightlessness would be counteracted by the nanomachines inside the space traveler's body. Presumably the nanomachines would also take care of any other problems, such as radiation damage or thus far unknown physical effects of prolonged space travel.

Another set of problems upon which nanotechnology can have only an indirect effect, is the unknown psychological problems of long term space travel. Being confined to a relatively small, unchanging environment with only a few other people for prolonged periods of time could lead to many sorts of problems. Various ameliorating factors exist. Virtual reality kinds of games and pursuits undoubtedly will become more sophisticated as our computing technology improves and could provide long term entertainment. More directly, the perfection of cryonics techniques would allow an interstellar traveler to simply go to sleep for extended periods of time and be awakened whenever there was an emergency or the destination was near.

Supplies for such a long journey should be no problem with the aid of nanotechnology. We already are capable of recycling a high percentage of air, water, and foodstuff. With the ability of nanotechnology to tear materials down atom by atom and rebuild needed molecules, food, pure water, and other materials would be assured. As long as the starship remains a closed environment, we should be able to achieve nearly one hundred percent recycling of the material it contains.

Of course, travel to other stars will not be everyone's cup of tea. The thought of isolation, the passage of many years back on Earth, and the simple dangers of the unknown will be sufficient to dissuade many, just as similar factors have dissuaded most in the past from exploring the Earth's surface. But the human race does produce those with motivation to become explorers and to probe the unknown regardless of personal danger or hardship, and undoubtedly that will continue to be so. And the stars will be the true final frontier for such people.

Meanwhile, without traveling to the stars, there will be plenty of opportunity for space exploration just within our own solar system. Mankind will most likely have some sort of presence on many of the planets and moons of the solar system. As mentioned previously, nanotechnology will make space travel extremely inexpensive. It will also make it much more comfortable for the traveler than it is currently. Without the prohibitive costs associated with current spacecraft, it will be possible to build large, luxurious spaceliners to ply the routes between the planets. Nanotechnology will also make it possible to build comfortable habitats in very hostile environments. Large scale terra-forming projects could potentially make Mars inhabitable by unprotected humans. Such a project might take several centuries, but with virtually unlimited life spans we can all well afford to wait.

Islands in Space

In addition to other planets and the moons of other planets in our solar system, habitations may be set up in the asteroid belt. Some of the asteroids are large enough to possess an appreciable gravity of their own. The most likely way to inhabit asteroids would be to hollow out the interiors and build living spaces in there.

A more common method of providing artificial habitations in space will be to build O'Neill-type structures (O'Neill, 1976). These habitations will be large hollow cylinders with interior worlds designed for human beings. The structures can be spun to provide gravity, and they will hold atmosphere, water, plants, and animals. They will be miniature Earths and will rely on solar power for their energy. They will be placed in stable fed with a slurry of the feedstock needed by the nanoassemblers inside the box to produce whatever is desired. Part of the feedstock materials for the nanoassemblers will come from highly efficient, on-site recycling. This recycling will be carried out by nanomachines which will disassemble discarded, worn-out and waste materials into their component atoms. As Drexler points out (1991), these habitations would also be built to include "smart" materials for all surfaces. These smart materials would incorporate nanomachines which would be programmed to keep the material clean at all times. Foreign substances would be disassembled and disposed of at the molecular level.

Clothing

The smart materials would include clothing. As mentioned briefly in the section on institutions and the demise of dry cleaners, clothing could also be manufactured to include nanomachines which would constantly maintain its integrity and cleanliness. They could also change shape, size, texture, feel, and color to accommodate the wearer. For those desiring to be provocative, areas of the garment could be programmed to randomly change in size, location, and transparency. Perhaps this feature could be under the conscious control of the wearer and be varied depending on the attractiveness of others in the environment.

orbits around planets, moons, the sun, and other places in-between. Different O'Neill habitats could be devoted to different purposes such as agriculture, manufacturing, various services, and the arts. They could also be havens for enclaves of the types discussed earlier where people of certain political, philosophical and/or religious beliefs could band together with their fellows and live according to their beliefs. They could structure their environment and their social and economic systems in such a way as to further and support those beliefs.

The materials to build these habitats need not be wrested from the Earth and brought up from its gravity well. Although the inexpensiveness of space flight made possible by nanotechnology would make such a method feasible, bringing in the material from the asteroid belt, the moon, or even the Oort Cloud would be more energy efficient. Though moving material from the Oort Cloud or the asteroid belt to Earth orbit would be a slow process, time will be relatively less important in the future. Thus, O'Neill type habitats can be built from raw materials which are plentiful in the solar system.

On a more grandiose scale, humans of the future might venture to build a Dyson sphere (Dyson, 1959). This would be an engineering undertaking of enormous magnitude. The basic idea of a Dyson sphere is to capture and utilize all of the energy emitted by a star. The way this is done is to enclose the star in a hollow sphere. The inner surface of the sphere, which is bathed by the energy of the star, is all inhabitable land. If you can imagine a sphere with a radius of one astronomical unit (the distance from the sun to the Earth, roughly ninety-three million miles) then you can imagine the awesome size of a Dyson sphere. The inner surface of the sphere would be about one billion times greater than that of the Earth. The materials could come from the astroid belt and planets. Since the Dyson sphere would have no gravity, another idea that has been suggested is to create a ring world around the sun and spin it to create gravity (Nichols, 1982).

Earth Transformed

But we've wandered rather far afield. This is just a glimpse of the kinds of space activities mankind might engage in in the future. By the time a person suspended now might be brought back, these possibilities will be enormous and complex and offer worlds of opportunity for exploration and living. Of course, Earth itself will also offer a future transformed by nanotechnology. Essentially the Earth will once again be the pristine environment it was for millions of years before man's industrial wastes began to transform and choke it. Nanotechnology, as described earlier, will allow us to clean up the excesses of the past from our land, water, and atmosphere. It will also allow us to support an extremely high energy, high abundance, high population society with no harm to the ecosphere.

Transportation

A major means of transportation could well be tunnels bored through the Earth by nanomachines and connecting many points. These tunnels could be created very efficiently and inexpensively and could be vacuumized and contain very high speed, magnetically levitated vehicles. With highly efficient solar power and nearly instantaneous communication from anywhere on the surface of the planet to anywhere else on the planet or in near Earth orbit, people may not be concentrated so highly in large urban environments. The necessity for clumping together for economic reasons will not be nearly as strong. People will tend to live in more dispersed patterns with a consequent improvement in life styles. Of course the locations where they live will enjoy blue skies, clean water and an unpolluted landscape.

Housing

With the availability of nanotechnology to produce goods inexpensively, housing will be large and elaborate compared to today's standards and will be filled with a cornucopia of material goods. Included in every household will be a nanotechnology manufacturing unit which would contain seed information for a wide range of products from appliances to clothing. The unit will be

> Being perfectly well dressed
> gives a feeling of tranquility
> that religion is powerless to
> bestow.
>
> Ralph Waldo Emerson
> (quoting a friend)

Life Cycles/Aging

And how will humans be changed in the world of your future? The basic subject of this book has been the profound changes nanotechnology will bring to the human condition, most profoundly, the prospect of immortality. Inherent in atomic level control of human cells is control over the aging process. Not only will we be able to halt the aging process in its tracks, but also to reverse it. This means that people will be able to choose, and change, their biological age at will. Apparent age will provide no meaningful clues to how long a person has been in existence. The most ancient of wisdoms may stroll in the guise of innocent youth. And that cantankerous white-haired gent may be a teenager exploring a territory that no longer exists except by choice. Profound changes indeed.

Not only will the end of life be changed, but also the beginning. The ways in which humans reproduce have been undergoing rapid change. Artificial insemination, fertilization of the egg outside the body, fertility enhancers which lead to multiple births, and the use of donor eggs are just some of the ways the birth process has been adapted to meet human needs. Nanotechnology will give us the power to take even more direct control over these processes. Control of the genetic information passed along to our offspring will allow precise choices over what are now the mostly random and dimly understood processes of inheritance. Natural childbirth will be but one of several choices for bringing new beings into the world.

To summarize then, the world of your future will be quite different from the present environment. That the differences will be as positive as the ones outlined above is almost guaranteed. Unless we have the kind of molecular control necessary to bring about these changes, you won't be awakened. The differences you can expect will be as profound as interstellar travel and immortality, and as mundane as programmable clothing next to your skin. Many additional living spaces for humans will be available, including those in space, on other planets, and in other stellar systems. The Earth itself should be transformed back into a near paradise. We will have more control over our environment, so much control that we'll no longer suffer from our abilities, but rather flourish because of them.

CHAPTER 23

Possible Serpents in Your Garden: Reasons for Living

> "Optimist" is what a pessimist calls a realist.
>
> Unknown

Well, I admit that the picture you paint of the possible future is very attractive. But don't you think you're being wildly optimistic that all those things might come to pass and that anyone around now will survive to see it?

Yes, perhaps a charge of optimism would be justified. As discussed in the section on decision making, it really depends on your subjective probability as to what is going to happen. If mine is substantially higher than yours, you might call me an optimist. Conversely, if mine is lower than yours, you would call me a pessimist. Part of the purpose of this book is to help you have an informed opinion about the likelihood that the events and changes described will happen. I hope that I have succeeded at least in giving you plenty of information to mull over.

The nature of the cryonics gamble, assuming you become suspended, is such that you are almost guaranteed awakening in the kind of world I have described *if* you are awakened at all. As discussed before, a number of elements will have to be in place for that awakening to be feasible. The technology will have to be available, and the world will have to be a place that will willingly support an additional population of those suspended. If the world has those kinds of capabilities, then the other features I have described, such as an abundance of material goods and inexpensive space travel, will be not only feasible but in place.

OK, so you're telling me that I would wake up in utopia, in heaven, that everything is going to be perfect, right?

No, I don't believe that. What one man has proposed another can fault. It's easy to think of ways in which the

world of the future will depart from utopia. To somewhat balance the picture, let's discuss a few of those possibilities. The starting point, of course, is that you are
awakened. The kinds of disasters and problems that
might prevent your successfully being awakened have
been covered and will not be talked about further here.

One category of things that might go wrong concerns
the misuses of nanotechnology which were discussed in
the "World of Slime" chapter. Just to refresh your memory, it is possible that you may awaken in a world that has
nanotechnology, but one in which, after you awaken,
things go radically wrong. In theory, nanoassemblers
could run wild and destroy the environment and all life
on Earth. We talked about how unlikely a scenario that is
because nanomachines need to be programmed and safeguards can be put in place to prevent them from exhibit-
ing any such dangerous abilities.

We also discussed the somewhat more likely deliberate
misuse of nanotechnology to create instruments of mass
destruction such as nanomachine plagues or of individual
destruction such as undetectable nanopoisons. Human
nature being what it is, these *are* possibilities and must be
addressed as the technology unfolds and develops.

The somewhat utopian picture of the future painted
in the last chapter was implicitly founded on the
assumption that our democratic institutions will prevail
in the age of nanotechnology. Another possibility for a
less than perfect world would be some sort of oppressive
dictatorship based on and supported by nanotechnology.

Thus far our democratic institutions have prevailed in the face of ever increasingly sophisticated technology, including nuclear power, and I see no reason to be pessimistic about that changing in the future. Clearly, though, that is one kind of change that could lead to a world much different from, and much less preferable to, the one described.

Let us assume stability in our political and environmental realities, and no sweeping danger from nanomachine plagues. There are still many possible ways in which the world of the future might deviate from perfection. One way has to do with our *raison d'etre*, reason for being. The general notion here has to do with the capability of nanotechnology to change the very fabric of our existence. Its capabilities are so broad and comprehensive and will change so many facets of our daily life that many of the things that motivate us to act, that occupy the hours and days and minutes of our lives, will no longer be in place.

Before going into detail about what I mean here, let me state a caveat. To some extent the point being made is comparable to our peasant of the middle ages speculating pessimistically about what he would do with his life if he had the advantages of modern civilization. If he didn't have to spend all day fetching wood and water and tilling his fields just to attend to his basic necessities, what could possibly occupy his time? What reason would he have for living? We're probably in that same situation in trying to speculate about the psychological realities of day-to-day life in the world of nanotechnology. Nevertheless, we can at least discuss how it will differ from our current situation.

We've already touched on the topic of careers. Obviously the upheavals which nanotechnology will cause in our institutions and organizations will make many kinds of jobs obsolete. These jobs give meaning to the lives of many people and also give them a way to occupy their time and to earn a living. It is equally obvious that nanotechnology and the opening of the space frontier will create many new and more interesting jobs. It is an open question as to whether these two factors will offset one another. In our current society automation is claiming a number of jobs, but is not generating a sufficiently large number of new, interesting, and well paid jobs to offset those losses. Too many of our new jobs are of the low-skill, minimum-wage type. There also seems to be a problem of adapting and improving the educational system to produce the kinds of workers needed by our evolving society. Nanotechnology may exacerbate this problem. On the positive side, though there will be dislocations, none of this will happen overnight. We will have time to prepare—too bad that's not one of our strengths as a species.

Equally troublesome are other kinds of activities with which humans occupy much of their time—sports and the performing arts in particular. Let's begin with sports. Think of what is entailed in someone excelling in sports and our fascination with them, whether we are fellow participants or spectators. Essentially great sports figures push the bounds of what is possible for humans. The incredibly acrobatic moves of a Michael Jordan, the strength and agility of a John Elway, the keen eye-hand coordination of a George Brett astonish us all. Now think about the capability of nanomachines to reconstruct our bodies closer to our heart's desire. Do you want denser bones, stronger muscles, faster reaction times, keener vision? All of these kinds of modifications will be possible with cellular level nanomachines to carry out the work. We've talked about their ability to repair, but obviously they also have the ability to enhance. If everyone can be enhanced, what then constitutes superior performance? Perhaps our abilities will still fall on some bell-shaped curve, but that is not clear from here.

The same sort of argument applies to the performing arts, such as dance and music. If a great set of vocal cords and powerful lungs are yours for the asking, who wants to listen to someone else sing? If your body can be enhanced to effortlessly perform the most difficult and graceful of ballet moves, what interest would you have in watching others? For that matter, how interested would you be in your own accomplishments if they were due not to talent and hard work but to nanotechnological modifications of your body?

Ah, you say, but it is more than simply the muscles and bones—it is a talent that expresses itself through the movements of the human body or the playing of musical instruments. I do not deny this, but let's carry these ideas to their logical extreme. If that talent can be recorded and captured as molecular changes in your brain as you perform, then it can be put on a computer chip and implanted and accessed by the brains of others. If you too could play a trumpet like Miles Davis or have at your fingertips all the chess strategies of the grand masters, what then will motivate you to get up every day?

Another type of danger altogether, previously mentioned, has to do with the power of nanotechnology to alter the mind, to operate on the pleasure centers, to become an addictive drug without parallel. Of course, some people currently have access to less powerful, but still very addictive drugs and take advantage of that. Presumably some percentage of the human population would continue to do so in the future.

All in all then the world of the future will not be utopian. The human race will still be striving to find its way in the universe. The material abundance we enjoy today is probably as immensely superior to that of our cave-dwelling ancestors as nanotechnological abundance will be compared to our current standards. The cave-dwellers did not live in utopia, we do not live in utopia, and the world of the future will not be utopia either. It will be, however, vastly different and vastly better.

CHAPTER 24

The Time of Your Life

> Too much of a good thing is simply wonderful.
>
> **Liberace**

And now it's up to you. At some point you will make a decision as to whether to pursue the ideas in this book. You will decide whether to take a shot at achieving personal immortality. You may do something immediately, or years from now, or never. Whatever you do, you will have made a decision. For now, let's play "what if." What if you do seek and gain immortality? What are your dreams, what will you do with yourself, how will you spend your time from here to eternity? It is important to remember that in judging the world of the future, one must be careful not to wear the blinkers of the past.

Would you want to travel? With the time available you could walk every square mile of the Earth's landmasses. You could travel to Earth orbit and visit the O'Neill habitats circling there. You could visit the moon. You could travel to other planets of the solar system. If you really like to travel, how would you like to visit another star and experience whatever marvels might be there? Perhaps you can be one of those to help answer the question as to whether or not there is life on other planets. If there is, what kind of life is it, how intelligent, how technically capable?

Maybe we can help those other life forms, if there are any, given our nanotechnology capabilities. This will bring up the interesting question of whether we *should* help even if we can. If there is no life on the planets you find, you can help transform a planet, make it capable of supporting life, human or newly created. Nanotechnology will make that possible. It will take a while, but you will have plenty of that commodity available. Or do you want to join the party at far edge of the galaxy after a truly epic journey of exploration?

Closer to home, how would you like to spend your time on Earth? What kinds of life experiences do you want to accrue? A career in science, in the arts, helping to heal mother Earth? How about all of those and any others that you can think of? Your future is wide open.

How about all those things you always wanted to learn but never had the time and energy for? Learn to play the piano, become a chess expert or a great chef, whatever your heart's desire. Or maybe you would like to worship Murtia, the goddess of laziness and languor. In an age of abundance mere survival should not be a problem. Try loafing for twenty years—see how you feel about it. You can always change your mind and become productive. Want to live for a while in a teeming metropolis full of cultural events and millions of people? Go do it. Or do you want to live with only the wind, the sun, and the stars for companions? Find that spot, live that life. Want to have a large family and preside over their tragedies and triumphs for many generations? You can do it. Dream whatever dream you can dream. Then make it come true.

As mortals we have always been condemned to live in only one era. You can read about life in medieval England, or see a movie about the old west, or speculate along with the anthropologists about the day-to-day existence of cultures long vanished. But there has never been a chance for anyone to actually live through and experience those kinds of sweeping changes. Although nanotechnology will usher in a new era, mankind will undoubtedly continue to change and grow far into the future. The difference is that this time you personally will be able to experience whatever lies ahead, for as long as you like.

The world of the future will be filled with many wonders, and challenges broad enough and deep enough to match the soaring spirit of an immortal population. I invite you to join me there.

Resources

KEY READINGS

Drexler, K.E. (1986) *Engines of Creation.* New York:Anchor Press/Doubleday.

Drexler, K.E., C. Peterson, and G. Pergamit (1991) *Unbounding the Future: The Nanotechnology Revolution.* New York:William Morrow.

Cryonics: Reaching For Tomorrow. (1993) Scottsdale, AZ: Alcor Life Extension Foundation.

KEEPING CURRENT

Alcor Phoenix
Focus: Cryonics: members newsletter
Eight issues/year
Alcor Life Extension Foundation
7895 E. Acoma Drive, #110
Scottsdale, AZ 85260-6916
800-367-2228
602-922-9013
$20/year

American Cryonics
Focus: Cryonics
Semi-annual publication
American Cryonics Society
P.O. Box 761
Cupertino, California 95015
408-446-4425
$35/year

Cryonics
Focus: Cryonics: general information
Quarterly publication:
Alcor Life Extension Foundation
7895 E. Acoma Drive, #110
Scottsdale, AZ 85260-6916
800-367-2228
602-922-9013
$15/year

Foresight Update
Focus: Nanotechnology
Semi-annual publication
Foresight Institute
P.O. Box 61058
Palo Alto, California 94306
415-324-2490
$25/year

The Immortalist
Focus: Cryonics
Monthly publication:
The Immortalist Society
24443 Roanoke
Oak Park, Michigan 481237
313-548-9549
$25/year

The Trans Times
Focus: Cryonics
Bimonthly publication:
Trans Time, Inc.
10208 Pearmain St.
Oakland, California 94603
510-639-1955
$12/year

Venturist Monthly News
Focus: Immortalist philosophy
Monthly publication:
Society for Venturism
10444 N. Cave Creek Rd.
Phoenix, AZ 85020
$12/year

CRYONICS ORGANIZATIONS

Alcor Life Extension Foundation
7895 E. Acoma Drive, #110
Scottsdale, AZ 85260-6916
800-367-2228
602-922-9013
Type: Non-profit, tax-exempt
Founded: 1972
Number signed up for suspension: 360
Number currently in suspension: 28
Initial membership cost: $150
Annual dues: $324
Full body suspension cost: $120,000
Neurosuspension cost: $50,000
Remote suspension capability: Yes. Initial suspension facilities in Florida and England, equipment and trained technicians in New York, Canada, Indiana, and Northern California. Remote recovery team will travel to death site and prepare patient for transport to suspension facility. Within 100 miles of Phoenix, or with special arrangements, the recovery team will come before legal death and standby to ensure the least delay between legal death and initiation of suspension.

American Cryonics Society
P.O. Box 761
Cupertino, California 95015
800-523-2001 / 408-734-4200

Type: Non-profit. Contracts with other organizations for services, BioPreservation, Inc. and the Cryonics Institute for suspension services, and the Cryonics Institute and CryoSpan Inc. for long term storage.
Founded: 1969
Number signed up for suspension: 100
Number currently in suspension: Some involvement with about 25
Initial membership cost: $376
Annual dues: $376 for three years, then $300/year
Full body suspension cost: Various options ranging from $37, 000 to $125,000
Neurosuspension cost: Various options ranging from $25,000 to $60,000
Remote suspension capability: Yes. The Society itself can provide the first stage of suspension in emergency situations, then contracted organizations take over.

CryoCare Foundation
P.O. Box 3631
Culver City, CA 90231
800-867-2273
Type: Non-profit. Contracts with other organizations for services, BioPreservation, Inc. for suspension services and CryoSpan Inc. for long term storage.
Founded: 1993
Number signed up for suspension: 100+
Number currently in suspension: None
Initial membership cost: $100
Annual dues: $350
Full body suspension cost: $125,000
Neurosuspension cost: $58, 500
Remote suspension capability: Yes, through BioPreservation, Inc.

Cryonics Institute
24443 Roanoke
Oak Park, Michigan 481237
313-548-9549

Type: Non-profit
Founded: 1976
Number signed up for suspension: 120
Number currently in suspension: 11
Initial membership cost: $1,250
Annual dues: $100 (not required)
Full body suspension cost: $28,000
Neurosuspension cost: Suspend only full body
Remote suspension capability: None

The International Cryonics Foundation
1430 N. El Dorado St.
Stockton, CA 95202
209-463-0429
Type: Non-profit. They function as trustees over the money set aside for suspension and long term care, and as patient advocates. The money is put into separate funds for each person.
Founded: 1990
Number signed up for suspension: 30 (suspensions conducted by other organizations such as Alcor and TransTime).
Number currently in suspension: None
Initial membership cost: $1000
Annual dues: $120
Full body suspension cost: Depends on suspension organization used.
Neurosuspension cost: Depends on suspension organization used.
Remote suspension capability: Depends on suspension organization used.

Trans Time, Inc.
10208 Pearmain St.
Oakland, California 94603
510-639-1955
Type: Commercial, for-profit
Founded: 1972
Number signed up for suspension: 40
Number currently in suspension: 9

Initial membership cost: None
Annual dues: $96
Full body suspension cost: $150,000
Neurosuspension cost: Do not perform neurosuspensions.
Remote suspension capability: None

INSURANCE AGENTS FAMILIAR WITH CRYONICS

Rich Balducci (WA residents only)
The Independent Order of Foresters
10107 S. Tacoma Way, Suite A-1
Tacoma, WA 98499
(800) 873-4463

Don Bannister
Independent Agent
2101 West Commercial Blvd., Suite 5100
Ft. Lauderdale, FL 33309
(305) 735 9000

Joseph Biggs (Century Insurance)
1700 W. Park Dr.
Westborough, MA 01581
(508) 836-4630

David M. Brandt
Wells Fargo Insurance Services
1000 Marina Blvd., 3rd Floor
Brisbane, CA 94005
(800) 255-2338

Jerr de Vaux, R.H.U., L.U.T.C.F.
50 Corporate Park
Irvine, CA 92714
(714) 660-1900

Robert A. Gilmore, Jr
Mary E. Naples, CLU
New York Life Insurance Company
4600 Bohannon Dr., Suite 100
Menlo Park, CA 94025
(800) 645-3338

Roger G. Hartman
Roger Hartman & Company
P.O. Box 3100
Evergreen, CO 80439
(303) 670-0054

Rudi Hoffman, CFP and Associates
1249 Robbin Dr.
Port Orange, FL 32119
(800) 749-3773

Abe Illowitz
New York Life Insurance Agent
340 Fifth Ave., Suite 2101
New York, NY 10018
(212) 502-3800

Mike Midlam, CFA
The Independent Order of Foresters
100 Border Avenue
Solana Beach, CA 92075
(619) 755-5151

Ed Muir (specializes in New York Life)
Muir Financial Services
11350 N. Meridian, #500
Carmel, IN 46032-4528
(317) 842-6233

Robert M. Rees
Robert M. Rees Insurance Agency
P.O. Box 42047
Oklahoma City, OK 73123
(405) 721-2021

Scott M. Russo (markets New York Life)
One American Place, Suite 800
Baton Rouge, LA 70825
(504) 387-0711

Bruce Schneider (specializes in Lincoln National)
718 NW 90th Terrace
Plantation, FL 33324
(800) 851-9033

Jim Yount
20200 Patric Court
Cupertino, CA 95014-44224
(408) 996-8710

INVESTMENTS

The Reanimation Foundation
Asset Preservation
16280 Whispering Spur
Riverside, California 92504
800-841-LIFE

References

Alkon, D.L. (1989) Memory storage and neural systems. *Scientific American.* July:42-50.

Biggart, M.J. and D.J. Bohn (1990) Effect of hypothermia and cardiac arrest on outcome of near-drowning accidents in children. *The Journal of Pediatrics.* 117(2-1):179-183.

Bridge, S.W. (1995) The legal status of cryonics patients. *Cryonics.* 16(1):4-11.

Clarke, A.C. (1994) 2001:The Coming Age of Hydrogen Power. *Cold Fusion.* 1(1):10-13.

Cooke, R.M. (1991) *Experts in Uncertainty: Opinion and Subjective Probability in Science.* New York:Oxford University Press.

Crick, F. and C. Koch (1992) The problem of consciousness. *Scientific American.* 267(3):153-159.

Cryonics: Reaching For Tomorrow. (1993) Scottsdale, AZ: Alcor Life Extension Foundation.

Drexler, K.E. (1986) *Engines of Creation.* New York:Anchor Press/Doubleday.

Drexler, K.E. (1988) Will change be abrupt? *Foresight Background.* 1:1-4.

Drexler, K.E. (1991) Molecular directions in nanotechnology. *Nanotechnology* 2:113-118.

Drexler, K.E. (1992) *Nanosystems: Molecular Machinery, Manufacturing, and Computation.* New York:John Wiley & Sons.

Drexler, K.E., C. Peterson, and G. Pergamit (1991) *Unbounding the Future: The Nanotechnology Revolution.* New York:William Morrow.

During, N. (pen name for Evan Cooper) (1962) *Immortality, Scientifically, Now.* (Privately published, reprint available through Alcor).

Dyson, F.J. (1959) Search for artificial stellar sources of infra-red radiation. *Science.* 131:

Eigler, D.M. and E.K. Schweizer (1990) Positioning single atoms with a scanning tunnelling microscope. *Nature.* 344:524-526.

Ettinger, R.C.W. (1964) *The Prospect of Immortality.* New York: Doubleday.

Fahy, G. (1991) A "realistic" scenario for nanotechnological repair of the frozen human brain. in *Cryonics: Reaching For Tomorrow* (see earlier reference).

FDA Consumer (1990) 24(7):19

Foresight Update (1995):20

Gershon, E.S. and R.O. Rieder (1992) Major disorders of mind and brain. *Scientific American.* 267(3):127-133.

Harris, S.B. (1989) Many are cold but few are frozen: a humanist looks at cryonics. *Free Inquiry* 9(2):19-24.

Henson, H.K. (1993) What to do with a million years. *Cryonics.* 14(7/8):12-13.

Lehninger, A. (1982) *Principles of Biochemistry*. New York:Worth.
Mergenhagen, P. (1991) Doing the career shuffle. *American Demographics*. 13(11):42-44.

Merkle, R.M. (1993) Estimates of technical success and survival strategies in cryonics. *Cryonics*. 14(9):16-17.

Merkle, R.M. (1994) The Molecular Repair of the Brain, Part I. *Cryonics*. 15(1):16-31; Part II. *Cryonics*. 15(2):18-30.

Nichols, P. (1982) *The Science In Science Fiction*. New York:Alfred A. Knopf, Inc.

O'Neill, G. (1976) *The High Frontier: Human Colonies in Space*. New York:William Morrow.

Perry, M. (1993) The first cryonics operation. *Cryonics*. 14(7/8):7-10.

Perry, M. (1994) The realities of patient storage. *Cryonics*. 15(2):8-10.

Platt, C. (1993) The Omni/Alcor Immortality Contest. *Omni*. 15(4):40-46.

Richardson, S. (1993) A violence in the blood. *Discover*. 14(10):30-31.

Roberts, K. (1978) *Society and the Growth of Leisure*. London:Longman Group Limited.

Rubenstein, E. (1994) Malthus does Cairo. *National Review*. 46:18.

Science and technology: a report to the President. (1993) *White House Office of Science and Technology Policy*.

Selkoe, D.J. (1992) Aging brain, aging mind. *Scientific American.* 267(3):134-142.

Sheskin, A. (1979) *Cryonics: A Sociology of Death and Bereavement.* New York:Irvington Publishers, Inc.

Smith, G.P. II (1983) *Medical-Legal Aspects of Cryonics: Prospects for Immortality.* Port Washington, New York:Associated Faculty Press.

Smith, G.P. II (1989) *The New Biology: Law, Ethics and Biotechnology.* New York:Plenum Press.

Storti, C. (1990) *The Art of Crossing Cultures.* Yarmouth, Maine: Intercultural Press.

Wikler, D. (1993) Brain death: a durable consensus? *Bioethics.* 7(2/3):239-246.

Zakharova, O.A. and V.P. Tumanov (1992) Time course of cessation of biosynthesis by brain cells after death. *Bulletin of Experimental Biology and Medicine.* 114(11):1706-1709.

Glossary

Atom: A unit of matter, the smallest unit of an element, having all the characteristics of that element and consisting of a dense, central, positively charged nucleus surrounded by a system of electrons. Atoms make up molecules and solid objects and are about a third of a nanometer in diameter.

Atomic force microscope: An instrument able to image surfaces to molecular accuracy by mechanically probing their surface contours.

Bacteria: Single-celled microorganisms about one thousand nanometers across.

Biostasis: A condition in which an organism's cell and tissue structures are preserved, allowing for later restoration by cellular repair machines. *Cryonic suspension* is a form of biostasis.

Cell: The smallest structural unit of an organism that is capable of independent functioning. The human body contains trillions of cells most of which contain all the organism's genetic information in the form of DNA.

Cellular Repair Machine: A system including nanocomputers and molecular-scale sensors and tools, programmed to repair damage to cells and tissues. A medical nanomachine.

Cryobiology: The science that studies the effects of low temperatures on living systems. Research in cryobiology has made possible the freezing and storing of sperm and blood for later use.

Cryogenics: The engineering science and technology of extreme low temperatures and their effects on physical systems and materials.

Cryonics: The practice of maintaining patients currently classed as legally "dead" at extremely low temperatures for treatment by the medical technology of the future.

Cryonic suspension: The process of cooling a human body to an extremely low temperature and the state maintained thereafter.

Cryoprotectant: A chemical inhibiting or reducing the formation of damaging ice crystals in biological tissues during cooling.

Culture shock: Feelings of depression, homesickness, distaste and sometimes fear caused by living in a foreign environment.

DNA (Deoxyribonucleic acid): A nucleic acid that carries the genetic information in the cell and is capable of self-replication. The protein molecules constructed from DNA information make up much of the molecular machinery of the cell.

Dyson sphere: A hollow sphere enclosing the sun at a radius of Earth's distance from the sun. The inner surface of the sphere would provide a living space a billion times larger than that of the Earth.

Genetic engineering: Scientific alteration of the structure of genetic material in a living organism.

Geometric growth: Growth occurring by some ratio, such as doubling or tripling, in a fixed period of time.

Information theoretic death: Irreversible loss of the structural information which encodes memory and personality. Also "memory" death.

Molecule: Group of atoms held together by chemical bonds; the typical unit manipulated by nanotechnology.

Molecular manufacturing: Manufacturing using molecular machinery, giving molecule-by-molecule control of products and by-products via positional chemistry. An application of nanotechnology.

Nano-: A prefix meaning one billionth (1/1,000,000,000). Nanotechnology operates at the nanometer scale, thus at a scale of one billionth of a meter.

Nanocomputer: A computer with parts built on a molecular, nanometer scale. A powerful nanocomputer will take up 1/1000 the volume of a typical cell and contain more information than the DNA in the cell.

Nanomachine: An artificial molecular machine of the sort made by molecular manufacturing.

Nanoseed: A unit of nanocomputers and nanoassemblers which, when placed in an environment containing sufficient raw material, automatically builds a pre-programmed structure or device.

Nanotechnology: Technology based on the manipulation of individual atoms and molecules to build structures to complex, atomic specification. Molecular manufacturing will be one important application of nanotechnology.

Neurosuspension: A cryonic suspension option in which only the brain, or the brain and head, is preserved. The technique rests on the assumption that cell repair technology will make it possible to generate a new body, to accompany the preserved brain, from the DNA code contained in brain cells.

Oort cloud: A very distant cloud of comet material surrounding the Sun beyond the orbit of Pluto.

Proximal probes: A family of devices capable of fine positional control and sensing, including atomic force and scanning tunneling microscopes. Proximal probes represent a possible path to nanotechnology.

Scanning tunneling microscope: An instrument able to image conducting surfaces to atomic accuracy. Has been used to create the letters "IBM" by positioning individual atoms.

Smart materials: Materials incorporating nanomachines and nanocomputers. These materials will be programmed to keep surfaces clean, respond to changes in the environment, and make complex changes on command.

Subjective expected utility (SEU): A formal model which can be used to help make important decisions. The model combines personal probabilities with personal judgments of worth, or utility, to evaluate the attractiveness of decision outcomes.

Index